How to Pass the RACP Written and Clinical Exams

How to Pass the RACP Written and Clinical Exams

The Insider's Guide

Second Edition

Zoë Raos
North Shore Hospital, Auckland, New Zealand

Cheryl Johnson
North Shore Hospital, Auckland, New Zealand

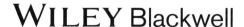

Registered Offices
John Wiley & Sons, Inc., 111 River Street, Hoboken, NJ 07030, USA
John Wiley & Sons Ltd, The Atrium, Southern Gate, Chichester, West Sussex, PO19 8SQ, UK

Editorial Office
9600 Garsington Road, Oxford, OX4 2DQ, UK

For details of our global editorial offices, customer services, and more information about Wiley products visit us at www.wiley.com.

Wiley also publishes its books in a variety of electronic formats and by print-on-demand. Some content that appears in standard print versions of this book may not be available in other formats.

Library of Congress Cataloging-in-Publication data applied for

ISBN: 9781118892633 [Paperback]

Cover image: Photograph taken by authors with permission from 3M Littmann Stethoscopes.
Cover design: Wiley

Set in 10/12pt WarnockPro by SPi Global, Pondicherry, India

Printed in Singapore by C.O.S. Printers Pte Ltd

10 9 8 7 6 5 4 3 2 1

The second edition is dedicated to Hector, Juno and Caleb.

Contents

Preface

'I take the view, and always have, that if you cannot say what you want to say in twenty minutes you ought to go away and write a book about it' (Lord Brabazon, 1884–1964)

After our group of registrars sat the RACP Written Exam in 2005 in Auckland, we thought back on how our lives had changed. Our houses were full of notes, textbooks and journal articles, and we were proud owners of impressive collections of highlighters. Our minds were full of little snippets of advice snatched in hospital corridors from our consultants and senior registrars: how to find old exam questions, how to sign up for courses and how to start a study group. After most of us passed the Written, we were compelled to write these snippets down so the collective wisdom could be passed on to the 2006 registrars. Then reality hit; there was another, harder exam to sit – the Clinical. Once again, we muddled through with an enormous debt to seniors who hauled us through short cases and long cases, gave us pep talks and lent us books. Many of us passed the Clinical Exam somehow. And what better way for us to continue the fine physicianly tradition of helping those who come after us than to write a book?

Ingrid and I, with the help of Pat Starkey, our editor with the patience of a saint, wrote *How to Pass* and published it through our local hospital. Our little book was well received and reprinted twice. Ingrid and I moved on to advanced training, fellowships, consultanthood and family life. Requests for copies of *How to Pass* kept popping up, and while there was content that remained relevant, it was time for an update. Ingrid passed the baton to me to update the book, which I have done with the help of Cheryl, some amazing guest star chapter authors (including paediatricians) and the current generation of exam-sitting registrars.

The journey through the RACP exams is long, arduous and, at times, painful. You'll laugh. You'll cry. You'll hurl. You'll lose some friends but make others. You will also gain a lot of knowledge, become a better doctor and before you know it, advanced training will be upon you, and your life as a physician or paediatrician will begin.

Take heart that you are not the first person to study for this 'quiz' and you won't be the last. With hundreds of hours of study, some personal sacrifice, advice that works and a spot of luck, we reckon you'll figure out How to Pass too.

Zoë Raos, Ingrid Hutton and Cheryl Johnson

About the Authors

Dr Zoë Raos, Author First and Second Editions

Gastroenterologist, General Physician and RACP Examiner
North Shore Hospital, Auckland, New Zealand

In 2005, Zoë was so convinced she'd failed her Written Exam that she jotted down some tips for the next attempt to help herself and anyone else the following year. She and her study group passed that year, they all passed the Clinical and have been friends ever since. She kept busy with advanced training in gastroenterology and general medicine, married Ben Hill and was involved in the RACP as chair of the College Trainees' Committee and Director of the Board. Zoë dragged Ben to England, did a fellowship at the John Radcliffe Hospital in Oxford in 2009 for a couple of years and returned (with a mind full of ideas, a passport with lots of stamps and a lovely little boy) to New Zealand for a consultant post at Waitemata District Health Board in Auckland. Zoë became an RACP examiner in 2016. Such is her dedication to this book, she wrote this bio three days before the birth of Juno, Hector's little sister.

Dr Ingrid Hutton (née Naden) – Co-Author of the First Edition

Rheumatologist, Coast Joint Care, Maroochydore, Australia

Ingrid sat and passed both sets of RACP exams in 2005 in Auckland. She now lives on the Sunshine Coast, Australia, with her husband, two kids and their dog. Ingrid works as a private rheumatologist which involves a lot of polypharmacy, social isolation and 'balancing the demands of competing medical conditions' (that phrase still comes in handy for GP letters). She doesn't miss doing weekend nights on call.

Dr Cheryl Johnson – Co-author of the Second Edition

Geriatrician and RACP Examiner, North Shore Hospital, Auckland, New Zealand

Cheryl passed the RACP Written and Clinical Exams in 2008. She spent the next five years in advanced training and became a geriatrician and general physician in 2013. Cheryl then overqualified herself as co-author by accepting a Geriatrician and Medical Tutor Specialist position at Waitemata District Health Board in Auckland. She is the RACP Director of Physician Education and is on the working group for the redesign of the Basic Training Curriculum. Cheryl has been an RACP examiner (NZ) since 2014 and organised the 2013 and 2015 Clinical Examinations at North Shore Hospital. She is the current chair of the Auckland Medicine Vocational Training Committee, the mother of Caleb who is at start school, uses her considerable charm to convince consultants to come in on Saturday mornings to tutor the candidates and is the adoptive big sister to all the trainees she whips into shape for these exams every year.

Acknowledgements

Many people have walked us through exams, advanced training, fellowship, motherhood and consultancy. We'd like to thank our friends, families, study groupies and fellow candidates. We couldn't have done it without you. We are eternally grateful to the patients and examiners who endured our practice cases – thanks for not laughing too openly at the time. We'd like to thank our colleagues, chapter authors and trainees who have been so generous with their input and contributions, be they emails, scribbles on napkins or chats in corridors. Your words of wisdom will smooth the path of those who follow. Thanks to our publisher for taking *How to Pass* to the next level and our wonderful families for teaching us about what matters in life every day.

While we can't list you all, there are some notable people who gave substantial time and advice for this book. Thank you for your contributions.

Chapter Co-Authors

Chapter 20 Suggested Approach to a Māori Patient in the Long Case – Dr Matthew Wheeler, Advanced Trainee, Dunedin

Chapter 30 How to Fail – The Outsider's Guide to the FRACP Exam – Dr Roderick Ryan, Paediatrician, Box Hill Hospital and Maroondah Hospital, Victoria, Australia

Chapter 32 Studying for the FRACP with a Family on Board – Dr Robert Wakuluk, Advanced Trainee, Auckland

Chapter 35 Preparing for Your Medical Interview – Dr Nalin Wickramasuriya, Paediatrician, Queen Alexandra Hospital, Portsmouth, UK

Significant Contributors

Dr Genevieve Ostring, Paediatrician and Clinical Examiner, Waitemata District Health Board

Dr Colette Muir, Developmental Paediatrician, Starship Hospital

Dr Stephen McBride, Infectious Diseases Physician, Middlemore Hospital

Dr Chris Hood, Renal Physician, Middlemore Hospital

Dr Mark Simpson, Neurologist, Auckland City Hospital and Waitemata District Health Board

Dr Diana McNeill, Endocrinologist, Middlemore Hospital

Dr Sophie Leitch, Advanced Trainee, Auckland

Dr Chloe Khoo, Advanced Trainee, Auckland

Dr Amanda Chen, Advanced Trainee, Auckland

Dr Michael Lee, Advanced Trainee, Auckland

Ms Pat Starkey, Clinical Education and Training Unit, Auckland City Hospital

Ms Gill Naden, Clinical Education and Training Unit, Auckland City Hospital

Dr Melanie Ang, Paediatrician, Middlemore Hospital

Dr Anthony Concannon, Paediatrician, Middlemore Hospital

Proceeds from the Authors' royalties will be donated to Autism New Zealand and the Children's Autism Foundation.

Illustrations

Diagrams, pictures and photographs by Zoë Raos

General Disclaimer

This book is littered with acronyms ranging from LFTs and ILD to RA and DLCO. We could have written the words all out in full but that would have taken us years and the book would have been enormous. We have worked hard to canvas as much advice from many registrars and consultants for both editions to reflect a range of successful approaches to the Written and Clinical Exams. There was not time to do a randomised double-blind placebo-controlled study on all the advice herein, so this book hovers above Z grade evidence with plenty of hearsay and rumour to further dilute the science. Please apply a large amount of common sense to your situation. If there is something earth-shatteringly awesome that helped you pass that is missing, please email us for the third edition. Our use of pronouns may also cause confusion. Usually, 'I' means 'Zoë' and 'we' can mean anything from 'Zoë and Cheryl', 'Ingrid and Zoë' to 'everyone we've talked to about this'.

Paeds Points

After many requests, we have added a paediatric flavour to the second edition and sincerely hope that paediatric registrars studying for their exams will find *How to Pass* to be more useful than before. After talking to some paediatricians about their own exam preparation, and what the current registrars do to get ready, we were pleasantly surprised how much similarity there is across both groups. For example, doing the hard yards for the Written and not annoying the examiners in the Clinical is the same. Please look out for Paeds Points for child health-specific information. If there are new and exciting developments in educational resources for paed trainees that we have not mentioned in this book, please contact us for the next edition.

Section 1

The Written Exam

1

Introduction to the Written Exam

Congratulations on embarking upon one of the most difficult but rewarding of career paths, that of internal medicine. Perhaps you see yourself as a budding neurologist or daydream about leading an adoring team on a fascinating general medical ward round. Maybe you will reach nirvana catheterising a left anterior descending artery. Maybe you enjoy working out a target weight for haemodialysis. Perhaps you've ruled out surgery (not crazy about detailing the boss's Audi), anaesthetics (big syringe, small syringe), radiology (too dark) and general practice (too general) and it comes down to internal medicine for adults or children. Internal medicine is not the career choice for everyone. The job of a long-suffering medical or paediatric registrar with the relentless on-call roster, permanent eye bags and a cynical outlook becomes even less attractive with exam stress. Please remember that you will be a consultant a lot longer than you will be a registrar. Your training will not last forever, so think of the career you want to have at the end of your training as well as the thorny and intense journey travelled to get there.

Historically, it has been rather straightforward getting a basic training post in medicine and paediatrics (a desperate phone call from the head of department the night before the job started worked for me). Times are changing. Before being eligible to even think about sitting the Written Exam, the trainee will need to have completed the requisite number of mini-CEXs and done some concerted navel gazing with the PREP programme. Paediatric trainees will have had a taste of exams with the Diploma. You may even have had (Shock! Horror!) an interview; if one is coming up then check out Chapter 35 for medical interview tips.

How to Pass the RACP Written and Clinical Exams: The Insider's Guide,
Second Edition. Zoë Raos and Cheryl Johnson.
© 2017 John Wiley & Sons Ltd. Published 2017 by John Wiley & Sons Ltd.

Upcoming changes
The FRACP Written and Clinical Examinations are held but once a year. It has been thus, despite conniptions, since the dawn of time. This book is written on the premise of an exam in February (for adult medicine); in fact, entire departments are aligned to this date like Stonehenge is to the solstice. There are plans afoot for a twice-yearly Written Exam. This is partially why old exam papers have been removed from the College circulation. We are not sure when this change will come, but there will be a transitional period between the old and new systems. Please keep your ear to the ground as this change may directly affect you.

Why Does The RACP Have a Written Exam?

The FRACP Written Exam is infamous for an enormous syllabus and intense focus on the minutest of details. The thought of this exam sends many prospective physicians packing to alternative careers. Another off-putting factor is that the examination, unlike many other specialties, is only held annually. High stakes. High stress. The preparation takes most candidates 8–12 months. Add study into the life of a busy medical or paediatric registrar and it is a miracle anyone sits at all.

While looking at old questions makes all newbie candidates clutch their heads in their hands, there is a method to the madness. The year of preparatory study lays the groundwork for advanced training, sharpens the mind, creates a robust knowledge base, increases confidence and improves performance at work.

The proportion of candidates passing the exam varies from year to year, and from region to region, but is generally above 50%. In the Auckland region, for example, the pass rate has risen from 50–70% a decade ago to over 80%. This means the majority of registrars, who commit to sacrificing almost a year of their life, put in the hard yards, work in a supportive hospital and revise properly, can hope to pass the Written Exam in their first attempt or, failing that, their second. Auckland paediatric trainees are even better off with a highly organised training programme, reflected in a 92% pass rate.

When is the Best Time to Sit?

Tricky. There is no perfect time in anyone's life. Candidates have sat (and passed) whilst heavily pregnant, newly postpartum, in the middle of house renovations, moving interstate and training for triathlons. Even so, it is crucial to weigh up the rest of your life goals before signing up.

A cautionary tale to those who have a burning desire to surge ahead and get that Written Exam over and done with as soon as possible. We have observed that candidates who allow for 1–2 years in addition to the minimum allowed by the College have an edge. These registrars handle work stress better, have more clinical experience to help with tricky and obscure Written Exam questions and perform to a higher standard for the Clinical Exam. Your registrar years will whizz by very quickly. Take another year now – no shame in it, might even do you some good. Also, once the exams are over, you want to be able to move straight into advanced training without having to spend another rotation doing more of the same work.

How Long Does It Take to Prepare for the Written Exam?

The exam is always in February for paeds and adult medicine. One year (i.e. starting in March the year before) is about enough time to get through the material. Some people start earlier, but find it difficult to keep up momentum. There are anecdotes of candidates who 'did no work until the November Sydney course' and passed, with tales of 'studying smart, not hard' – we don't believe them! The Law of Mass Effect states the harsh truth – the more time you put in, the more you learn. In Chapter 3 we will give some pointers to efficient and effective revision. This is a high-stakes, high-calibre examination. Give yourself plenty of time to prepare.

Am I Ready to Sit This Exam?

If you're not sure that you want to sit just yet, consider sitting in with an existing study group and see how you fit. Canvas opinion from local registrars who have passed (and failed) recently. Finally, if you're still in a quandary, it can be useful to ask your ward consultant or educational supervisor if he or she thinks you're ready. Once you have decided to sit then the best approach is to hurtle wholeheartedly into revision. The best strategy is to commit to sitting, work hard and pass the first time. Candidates with multiple half-hearted unsuccessful attempts are even more distraught than those poor souls who slog their guts out, have a bad exam day and fail. If you haven't made your mind up by July whether to sit the following year, leave it for another year as there may not be enough time. There is no shame in this decision and it will probably pay off, as that extra year will mean more experience (as long as the procrastination ends eventually!). Remember – better to sit once and sit well.

Decision Made. Sitting the Written

Congratulations! You are not put off! It is important to know what you're up for. Before we embark on the intricacies of how to pass, may we introduce you to the exam itself.

How Does the RACP Write the Exam and Come Up With All Those Questions?

Without giving away trade secrets, we will attempt to describe how the exam is set. Knowing how the exam is written helps you tackle it. There are four RACP exam committees.

- Adult Medicine Written Exam Committee
- Adult Medicine Clinical Exam Committee
- Paediatric and Child Health Written Exam Committee
- Paediatric and Child Health Clinical Exam Committee

The two Written Exam Committees do things slightly differently but the overall premise is the same. Both committees have representatives from every medical subspecialty known to the College/humanity. Each member of the committee formulates a number of questions that they think should be included in the exam. Other College fellows are able to submit questions also. The committees meet and all submitted questions are reviewed and agreed upon, revised or rejected. By September of the prior year, the exam is set in stone. So anything in a journal after the end of September is unlikely to be examined.

The brief of question writers is to come up with an MCQ that is set at the level of a trainee at the end of basic training. Not a subspecialist. Not even advanced trainee level. For example, you are not expected to know every single monoclonal antibody in existence, but it is fair game to be asked about the complications of TNF inhibitors.

For those who have sat the exam before, or who have already started studying, you may be quietly laughing (or perhaps crying) to yourselves at the thought of that last question you spent four hours trying to solve being allegedly set at basic trainee level.

Structure and Schedule

Here is the format of the exam. It is the same for paediatrics. It is worth noting that, especially in Paper 1, questions can be very similar if not identical across the adult medicine and paediatrics papers.

> **Morning**
> Paper 1 – Medical Sciences: 70 questions; time allowed: 2 hours
> **Lunch break** (where no-one really eats that much)
> **Afternoon**
> Paper 2 – Clinical Applications: 100 questions; time allowed: 3 hours

Most questions are in **A-type multiple-choice format**, meaning the candidate chooses the single best answer of the five options given, and shades the appropriate box on a separate answer sheet.

In Epstein–Barr virus infection, which one of the following peripheral blood cell types would most likely contain the virus?

A Neutrophils
B Atypical mononuclear cells
C Monocytes
D T cells
E B cells

Answer: E

Since 2013, **extended matching questions** (EMQs) have been included in the exam. Several questions (each worth one mark) based around a theme are bunched together and organised into three parts. The first part is an option list of eight possible answers. The second part is a lead-in statement. The third part has the stems (the actual exam questions) as clinical vignettes. To answer each exam question, the candidate works backwards: reads the vignette, keeps the lead-in statement in mind, then chooses the correct answer from the option list. Each correct answer scores one mark and an incorrect answer zero. Confused? Best to go through an example.

Option list

A Aortic dissection
B Ankylosing spondylitis
C Lumbar spondylosis
D Metastatic malignancy
E Vertebral fracture
F Prolapsed intervertebral disc
G Intervertebral disc infection
H Pars interarticularis defect

For each patient with back pain, select the most likely diagnosis.

Stem

1 A 35-year-old man has an eight-month history of lower back pain predominantly in the central lumbar region and left buttock. His pain is worse in the morning and there is some improvement during the day. On examination, there is restriction of all spinal movements and tenderness over the left sacroiliac joint.

   Answer: B

2 A 29-year-old woman presents with sudden-onset low back pain. She describes her pain as constant in nature and not affected by posture or movement. On examination, all spinal movements elicit pain. She had been treated for a urinary tract infection two weeks prior with a course of norfloxacin.

   Answer: G

How Does the College Decide Who Passes and Who Fails?

Your papers are handed in, the candidates collectively collapse in an exhausted heap, then the papers are marked electronically. It is not quite as simple as one correct answer = one mark chalked up. Some questions are flagged as 'good discriminators' by a complicated actuarial equation. If the vast majority of candidates get a question correct or incorrect, it is chucked out as being a poor discriminator. This usually applies to repeated questions from past exams. Questions that discriminate between the highest and the lowest candidate scores are given more weight. After more statistical jiggery-pokery, the candidates are ranked in order, a percentage pass mark is decided upon and a line is drawn between successful and unsuccessful candidates. At least, that's our understanding of the whole thing.

Finally, whether you pass or fail, the College sends you a post-mortem of your exam with your marks for each paper and ranks you against all the other candidates. This information is for your eyes only – no one else receives it and you can choose to burn it once you have read it!

We have included a past candidate's results statement as an example.

RESULTS STATEMENT
FRACP Written Examination: March 2014

Name:

FRACP ID:

Your Overall Score and result: **96** **Pass**

Pass Mark for the examination: **92**

Paper 1 (Medical Sciences): **34** (Maximum score is 60)
Paper 2 (Clinical Applications): **62** (Maximum score is 90)

The figure below shows the range of scores in this examination. The passing score and the average score are marked and your score is indicated by the arrow.

The figure below shows the range of scores for Medical Sciences and Clinical Applications in this examination. The score ranges obtained are indicated by the shaded regions. Your scores are indicated by arrows and the average scores are shown with lines.

Your subspecialty scores:

	Number of questions	Correctly answered		Number of questions	Correctly answered
Cardiology	11	7	Infectious Diseases	9	7
Clinical Epidemiology	5	1	Intensive Care Medicine	7	6
Clinical Genetics	6	4	Medical Oncology	8	6
Clinical Pharmacology	6	4	Nephrology	10	8
Dermatology	0	0	Neurology	12	9
Endocrinology	10	7	Palliative Medicine	0	0
Gastroenterology	12	8	Psychiatry	6	2
Geriatric Medicine	10	8	Rheumatology	9	6
Haematology	11	6	Thoracic Medicine	9	3
Immunology & Allergy	9	4			

Not official unless issued without alterations

Results Statement

Summary

- Our dear College works hard to make exam questions of a good standard and at the level of a trainee at the end of basic training.
- The Written Exam is actually two exams on one day. What a day!
- There are two types of question: A-type and EMQ.
- It takes a year to prepare.
- If you're tempted to sit the exam with bright-eyed and bushy-tailed enthusiasm shortly after starting basic training, think again. Allowing an extra year is almost always the right choice.

2

Preparation

One Year Out – What to Do Before You Even Start Studying

Before you open a book or look at an MCQ, we suggest getting some essential jobs done first. We have observed several pre-studying strategies that successful candidates have in common.

Check Eligibility to Sit

Make sure you've ticked all the boxes for PREP with the RACP so that a year of hard work is not thwarted for the sake of a missing mini-CEX.

Make the Decision to Sit by March the Year Before

Alternatively, make the decision not to sit, be glad you didn't and enjoy your year of freedom. We labour this point for good reason: it is indecision that has killed the possibility of passing for many candidates, as they flounder about for six months, sometimes committed to studying, sometimes not. If you've not started studying by June, it is far too late. Make an active decision.

Fill in All the Necessary Paperwork So You Can Sit the Exam

This seems obvious but some candidates have studied hard until November, then discovered too late that they are not eligible to sit. Don't let this be you! Fill in the forms and check with your Director of Physician Education.

How to Pass the RACP Written and Clinical Exams: The Insider's Guide,
Second Edition. Zoë Raos and Cheryl Johnson.
© 2017 John Wiley & Sons Ltd. Published 2017 by John Wiley & Sons Ltd.

Form a Study Group

From our observation, this will increase your chance of passing so much that we have dedicated Chapter 5 to it.

Book Well Ahead into a Two-Week Exam Preparation Course

These well-run courses are hosted for adult medicine trainees in Dunedin, Sydney and Melbourne and for paediatric trainees in Auckland and Sydney roughly four months before the exam. They are an excellent way to consolidate knowledge, give a boost of momentum and get the candidate used to exam conditions two-thirds of the way through your preparation. Exam courses are covered in detail in Chapter 8, including for paediatric trainees. Secure a spot.

Organise Study Leave and Annual Leave

Get these organised well in advance with your hospital, including the days leading up to the exam. You may need to do swaps with other registrars to get out of night duty on the night of the exam or to get to a study course. This is better done now, as the last three weeks before the exam is the worst time to ask for favours! For study leave, most candidates find 4–5 single weeks spaced over the year, plus two weeks off for a revision course, works well. You only have a finite amount of study leave so allow for some to cover the Clinical Exam. Make sure you plan for breaks and holidays too. Don't take so much leave that your rotation can't be accredited by the College. It's a balancing act.

Try to Find an Exam-Friendly Job

Some jobs are incredibly busy, with 0% chance of getting to teaching. Some are so cruisy your brain turns to mush. There is no perfect job for passing this exam, but ask around about jobs with high pass rates, forgiving rosters and the possibility of taking study leave. Consider a job share with a fellow sitter, if you can afford the drop in pay, but check it is allowed in your centre before setting your heart on it.

Almost more important than a relaxed timetable are two other things – first, proximity to peers in the same boat and second, the quality of FRACP teaching. Some hospitals are incredibly well organised with access to lectures, protected teaching time, extra tutorials and clinical teaching. This is not restricted to big academic centres; there are many smaller hospitals across Australia and New Zealand with an outstanding track record in supporting their trainees through their FRACP exams, and this is reflected in their pass rates.

Prepare the Team at Home

Explain to your family and friends that you are becoming a self-imposed slave to the Written Exam. This is a tough exam that will require a lot of your time and energy, and support (be it moral or practical) is crucial. Do not take the support of your loved ones for granted – put in some effort to maintain relationships. If you have children, this will be really hard on you, and them. Plan fun things to do, and include family time in your study timetable. Use this as a reward for study sessions. And remember, by passing this exam you are advancing your career, so you are better able to provide for your family. Please check out Chapter 32 for more tips on studying when there are ankle biters in the house.

Prepare the Team at Work

Explain to your house officer and boss that you need to be freed from duties when at all possible for teaching sessions and lectures. Apologise in advance for the grumpiness that will come as the exam draws ever nearer. Regular bribes of coffee and cake can grease the wheels. Your boss will have endured exams, and will hopefully understand. Your juniors will be looking ahead to their own career paths, and will hopefully take this as an opportunity to step up. Remember that you are an employee and a colleague; there is a delicate balance between assertively getting to teaching while leaving your patients and juniors organised with clear plans, and aggressively skiving off to the library before the ward round with ill-prepared patients and furious colleagues. Generally speaking, medical and paediatric registrars are a dedicated bunch who could take a lesson from their surgical colleagues in asserting their right to attend teaching, but there are a few who take the proverbial.

Get a Mentor

Find someone friendly from the previous year from whom to cadge lecture notes/old exams/material from course/tips. They will surely be delighted to offload five boxes of material to weigh down your bookshelves in lieu of theirs.

Organise a Study Space

Set aside a pleasant place at home with a desk, decent chair, a good lamp and logical storage for the phenomenal amount of written material you will receive and generate, even in the electronic age. Many candidates need a change of scene and prefer the library, but you still need somewhere to keep all the guff.

Prepare Yourself and Make an Overall Plan for the Year

This is the hardest task by far. Have your eye on the prize, and take time to plan the attack. A wall planner is useful, as is setting goals for the overall study plan. Decide on your approach (see Chapter 6 for wallpapering your mind) and accept that your goals will shift as the year progresses.

Summary

- The best way to pass this exam is to make the commitment to pass and stick with it.
- Carefully consider when is the best time for you to sit this exam. The best time is not always the soonest time.
- Fill in all the paperwork so you are eligible to sit.
- Get a study group together.
- Book leave in advance, and sign up for a two-week course.
- You, those around you and the place you will study all need to be prepared.

3

How to Start Studying for the Written Exam

This chapter includes concepts and ideas from a book called *Managing your Mind*, by Hope and Butler.[1] It covers much ground, including time management, relationships, how to study, how to recover from depression. I wish I'd known about this book before I started studying for the exam. In fact, this book should be handed out to everyone at high school. It is a well-written self-help book grounded in quality evidence and good practice, and my enthusiasm for it knows no bounds. Short of reprinting the entire text, we've included key strategies along with tips from registrars past and present to help you study, and remain relatively sane.

How to Manage Your Time

To manage time, you must manage tasks. By understanding the nature of these tasks and learning how they affect each other, time can be freed up, even for a time-poor medical or paediatrics registrar working 70 hours a week. The premise – every task we do in life can be placed into one of the four sectors of this pie chart (adapted from *Managing Your Mind*).

If you always find yourself spending your precious time on tasks you wish you didn't, with no time to study, relax or enjoy yourself, an excellent exercise is to collect your own data for a few days by writing down what you do and how long it takes. Your data will be affected by observer bias, but it will still give you a greater understanding. Here are examples of different kinds of tasks (see fig (a)).

---

1 Butler, G and Hope, T. (2007) *Managing Your Mind – the mental fitness guide*, 2nd edition. Oxford University Press. ISBN: 9780195314533

How to Pass the RACP Written and Clinical Exams: The Insider's Guide, Second Edition. Zoë Raos and Cheryl Johnson.

(a) Understanding Different Tasks

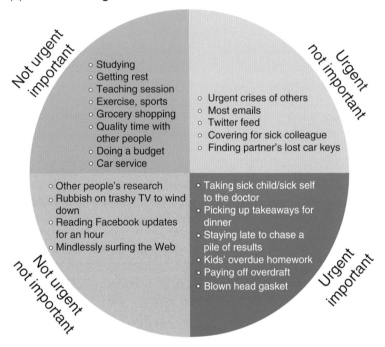

Urgent and Important

Anything that just can't wait. Getting sick and going to the doctor, staying at work late to chase a pile of overdue results, spending an hour getting the power turned back on as the electricity bill wasn't paid, picking up takeaways for dinner at 9 pm or missing study group to do slides for grand round. A mechanical metaphor: driving your car with smoke pouring out of the bonnet for a blown head gasket as no one has put coolant in the engine for months.

Urgent and Not Important

Usually, these tasks are meaningful to other people, mean little to you but just have to get done by someone. For example, missing a teaching session to do a family meeting as your house surgeon is sick, an ED nurse paging you about a discharge summary that needs to be done by another team, doing a talk for your boss as she will be at a conference. A mechanical metaphor: driving someone else's car with a flat tyre to the repair shop, then the cops give you a ticket for an expired registration.

Not Urgent and Not Important

These tasks seem compelling at the time and then you kick yourself afterwards. Watching rubbish on telly, mindlessly surfing the internet or social media. A mechanical metaphor: spending three hours deciding what colour of fluffy dice to hang from the rear vision mirror.

Not Urgent and Important

These are the tasks that we want to do but never seem to have enough time in the day to get done. Some examples – studying, exercise, getting a flu jab, grocery shopping, making healthy meals and putting them in the freezer, seeing friends, taking kids to the park, watching a programme on telly that you are really looking forward to, sending an email to a mentor, doing a budget and going to study group. A mechanical metaphor: taking your car in for a service and oil change, and having the nice surprise that someone has cleaned it.

Beyond the crazy hours we work, and the demands of training and exams, doctors are historically hopeless at task management outside work. We are time poor, really good at helping other people and thrive on last-minute deadlines. We take on urgent and unimportant tasks, mistaking them for proper emergencies. Many doctors are also aces at mindless activities that are neither urgent nor important, as they seemingly help us to zone out and wind down after a crazy day. Not urgent but important tasks like exercise and study get shunted. So, our week might look something like this fig (b).

No wonder registrars feel physically ill at the thought of finding time to study. On this pie chart, there is barely enough time to pee let alone go to study group. Do not despair! What is the purpose of this exercise? Hope and Butler state that the ultimate idea (within reason) is to know who you are, and what is important to you, then get rid of everything that is not important. This frees up time for the important stuff – which is not only study but other things like spending time with people you care about.

The next massive mind-change that will help your time management for the better is to spend *as much time as possible on non-urgent, important tasks.* By doing this, you will actually take tasks straight

(b) **Crises Prevail**

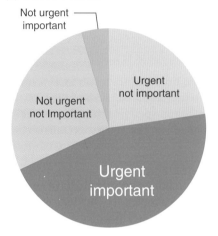

Urgency overwhelms everything. Important tasks like study and relaxation get shunted into the background. Fast track to stress and disorganisation.

out of the 'urgent' pile (think of the analogy of the blown head gasket versus taking the car in for a service). Stress levels drop and life becomes much more manageable. Your pie chart could look something like this.

Non-urgent, important tasks include leisure, study, exercise, relaxation and time off. It is important to realise that relaxing purposefully by reading a novel, taking your kids to a movie or going to yoga is different from those inane, non-urgent, not important weaselly time wasters (social media, bad TV ...) that we all mistake for relaxation. Also, there will always be genuine emergencies; the trick here is to see the difference between urgent, important emergencies and tasks that are only urgent because someone else says they are, or tasks that are forced into urgency by your own procrastination. Learning to turn down non-urgent non-important tasks is key to giving more time to important things. Another way to free up time is outsourcing to someone else's pie chart. Cleaners, online grocery shopping, healthy meal delivery and asking your partner or parent to help with the children's homework are all ways you can free up a bit of time. Specifically, as we will discuss, 35 minutes at a stretch for a productive study session fig (c).

(c) **Productivity Prevails**

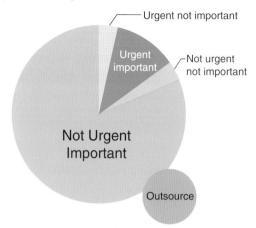

Productive task allocation means study can actually happen.
This requires a leap of faith -to spend more time on non-
urgent but important tasks so less crises happen.
Outsourcing helps.

While it would be lovely if everyone subscribed to our personal world-view as to what is crucial and what is irrelevant, for better or worse we live in a world with other individuals, complete with their own demands and ideas. Clashes occur when a problem that is terribly urgent and important to someone else is neither urgent nor important to you. This causes frustration as two individuals can have differing perspectives and needs. Communication and negotiation is the next step. Let's step in to a common clash as the department secretary angrily shoves a massive pile of overdue dictation into your arms while you are running out the door to get to teaching. If you do the dictation now, you miss teaching and that is terrible for you. If you ignore her and walk out, she will be furious and tattle to your boss – terrible for you too. How can this situation best be handled? Here's what you could say to the secretary:

'I can see that this pile of dictation is really urgent, and it sure is important to you and the patients to get this done. Look, I have to leave the office right now for a teaching session for my big exam in four weeks. I don't want to miss the bus so I need to leave right now. I will come into work early tomorrow morning and get the dictation done first thing. Is that OK? Then the dictation is done in good time for you, and I get to teaching.'

That's better. The secretary feels her request has been listened to, you've negotiated a reasonable compromise and (urgently and importantly!) you are getting to your teaching session on time. Understanding the different motivations and priorities of other people demonstrates insight and maturity, is a key skill to performing well in a long case, and essential to being a successful physician, paediatrician and human being.

Dealing with Stress

Yerkes and Dodson were forward-thinking psychologists. Their law from 1908 essentially states that, without stress, nobody would do anything. The performance of difficult or complex tasks then increases with stress in a linear fashion to a sweet spot. This makes sense – as exams draw closer, the pressure comes on and the brain kicks into gear like a well-oiled machine. But our brains can only handle so much stress. Piling on the pressure beyond the sweet spot will plateau your performance as stress keeps escalating with increasing fatigue. It gets worse. The performance plateau cannot be sustained with ever-increasing stress – performance then *slides* precipitously, all the way to burnout (see fig (d)).

(d) **The Stress Performance Curve**

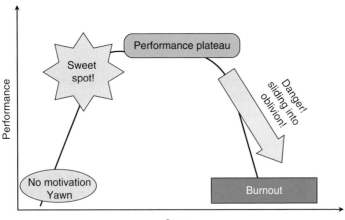

We are all different in the amount of stress we can handle, and very different in our perception of the pressure we are under. Many doctors have no insight that their performance is slipping as the stress piles on. Some individuals are able to absorb a lot of stress and maintain peak performance whilst others slide into fatigue and burnout oblivion. For medical and paediatric registrars, handling stress is part of a very demanding job. Studying for such a difficult exam adds considerable stress, and pushes us away from the sweet spot into the performance plateau. We all have our limits. We tip easily to oblivion, finding ourselves crabby, irritable and far less resilient at handling the knocks that life and work throw at us. Then, our ability to study evaporates, adding more stress. While this can be a lesson learned the hard way, there is much to be done to reduce (not eliminate) stress in life, work and study. It is possible to drag oneself back from burnout to the sweet spot. It is far better to be insightful and aware of increasing stress. Look back at the curve. When the pressure gets too much, *reducing* your stress will *increase* your performance. It is a proven fact. Build relaxation and self-awareness into your study routine and you will study more effectively (and be a happier person).

Advice from Registrars on Studying and Keeping Sane(ish)

These are quotes and bits of advice we've saved up over the years from many registrars. Most advice falls into two groups: time management and Jedi mind tricks.

- Accept the inevitable – this is going to be a tough year. Be kind to yourself.
- Sleeping and eating properly are very important
- You may gain 5+ kilos. You may also lose 5+ kilos. Try not to worry about the kilos too much.
- **Not studying is worse than studying.** We were paralysed by a fear of failure at times, struck down by anxiety. Sometimes the best thing to overcome that fear is a short, sharp study session to keep up momentum and morale.
- A fit body = a fit mind. Keep up regular exercise by going to the gym, playing sport or walking your dog.

- Have at least one clear night or entire day off a week (e.g. Friday). Go to the movies, do cross-stitch, go rock climbing, whatever works for you.
- Do not feel guilty if you have a day off. In fact, if you're in a total study funk then a day or weekend, sometimes even a week off, can be the best thing you can do to gain some perspective, as long as you can get going again. We all had time off studying leading up to the exam. At least have Christmas or your cultural equivalent off.
- If you find yourself rocketing along and down the stress/performance curve, recognise this before you slip to oblivion. It is difficult (not impossible, but difficult) to recover from burnout with an exam deadline looming.
- If you're stuck, then do something different. Old questions, MKSAPs or the Harrison's MCQ book are handy when you just can't stand reading another review article. Do a few questions, look up the answers and learn something. Get the study group together and refocus.
- Overall, the general rule is to be the tortoise, not the hare. Start early. It may not seem like it but the hour you do at home each night after work while you're missing bad telly really adds up in the long run.
- When we started studying, we couldn't sit still for more than five minutes. It took a long time to be able to concentrate for an hour. Start low, go slow.
- Get rid of as many distractions as you can. There are cool web-based programs that can lock you out of Facebook and Webmail for certain periods of time. Turn off your phone. Make the most of that precious hour you have freed up.
- Some (highly competitive, went to private school) people claimed to study for 10 hours every day. The majority of us could manage two hours after work and 3–4 hours on days off at the most. Concentration ability increases as the exam draws ever nearer.
- Time off is really important. Reward yourself with relaxing and socialising activities.
- Keep healthy by reducing alcohol and eliminating other harmful substances
- **You will not know everything** regardless of the amount of study you do. You will also find you forget things a few days after studying them! The memory is a strange place. Regular revision of work you have done before will help cement things in your mind.
- We found having a timetable for the year essential. The syllabus is vast and the temptation is to keep going on one subject until you

'really understand it'. Unfortunately, this technique usually results in you getting bogged down on the first subject and forgetting to move on to anything else. Without some sort of timeframe to keep you moving, you risk getting to the final week and finding you still have to cover all of endocrinology, respiratory, ID, statistics and pharmacology in two days!

- Organising study material is essential. You will be inundated. Most people used big folders, one per topic. Be organised with your computer/Dropbox files too. File everything as you go to avoid the fire risk from piles of stuff all over your house.
- Be co-operative with the other people studying from your hospital. Share information with one another. Tell each other what is helpful. Hoarding secret piles of resources will not make the difference between passing and failing but it will lose you friends. Some registrars set up a generic Dropbox account to disseminate helpful articles, study guides and answers to obscure questions. Share with others, and others can share with you.
- Studying is hard on those around you (partners, flatmates, whanau). Thank them regularly for their tolerance.
- **Your learning needs to be active.** Unlike Neo from *The Matrix*, you cannot plug a cable into the back of your head and suddenly become a kung fu master or (more usefully for most of us) an immunologist. Most people need to take notes, summarise, do mind maps as they read or the information doesn't enter the brain.
- Once you've decided which resources to revise (this took us about a month!) then you **just have to start.** At page one, or the subject that everyone in your group wants to go over. It doesn't matter where you start, just don't procrastinate too long.

A plea …

If you, like many doctors before you, feel yourself slipping into depression, anxiety or substance addiction (or find yourself on the wrong side of any parts of the DSM 5), please seek help urgently. This exam is important, but not as important as you. Take the time you need to heal, and seek expert advice. Some find study to be quite therapeutic, and part of the routine of getting better. Some need to focus on themselves, get serious help and defer the exam for 12 months. Your health and happiness trump all else.

Evidence-Based Study – Break It Down!

Much research has been done about how humans efficiently lay down memory. Oh, how we recall our inefficient student days, hours spent in the Philson Library, drinking Red Bull and continuously studying for hours on end until the librarians strong-armed us out the door, twitching, hungry and delirious. Once again, *Managing Your Mind* has come to the rescue. We now know that breaking down study time into bite-sized chunks is effective, and trains your memory. This general principle is also espoused by a very simple, widely used 'Pomodoro Technique', in which 25-minute work intervals (timed on a tomato-shaped kitchen timer, hence 'pomodoro') are used to maximise efficiency and manage distractions (http://pomodorotechnique.com/). Breaking down study into chunks means new memories are effectively laid down, whilst medium-term memories are condensed and consolidated. We wish that someone had advised us about how to make our memory work *before* we sat this exam. Let our loss be your gain.

This is one way you can organise your study structure into bite-sized chunks that will maximise your memory's capacity fig (e).

20 minutes studying a new topic
3 minutes tea break or rest
3 minutes revising a topic from yesterday
3 minutes revising a topic from the previous week
3 minutes revising a topic from last month
3 minutes revising the new topic again
=35 minutes study time

(e) Studying in Bite Sized Chunks

20 mins	3 min	3 min	3 min	3 min	3 min
New Study – topic 1	Tea break	Yesterday's topic	Last week's topic	Last month's topic	Today
New Study – topic 2	Tea break	Yesterday's topic	Last week's topic	Last month's topic	Today
New Study – topic 3	Tea break	Yesterday's topics	Last week's topic	Last month's topic	Today

Have another little rest, then repeat with a new topic.

The 'New Study' can be flexible – perhaps listening to a podcast, doing one or two MCQs and looking up the answers, reading a review article, going over study notes or lecture slides. A quick break, then the remainder of the session is spent sequentially revising topics from the previous day, week and month, each time laying down memory. This latter time is not wasted. The evidence tells us to resist the temptation to only look at new material, as regular revision is what really makes the material stick. We postulate that variations of this study technique is why parents often pass this exam – with strictly limited time, any study done is effective and efficient by sheer necessity.

However you study, your ability to concentrate will improve as the months go by. We remember those first frustrating months of being unable to sit still at a desk for 15 minutes, then fidgeting our way to the kettle. You're training your brain for a marathon, so be easy on yourself.

What About Taking Notes?

Writing whilst studying increases concentration and productivity. The notes can act as a useful memory aid for future revision sessions, and making notes gives a sense of achievement. Notes can be written in the margins of articles, highlighted in books with annotations, typed and saved on a computer or hand written on paper or little cards. Whatever way you write notes, make sure they are organised and filed to avoid wasting time. A minority of candidates insist that making notes is a waste of time – they may have photographic memories or have a different learning style that lays down memories and facts differently. For the vast majority, making notes is an essential part of study.

Getting Down to Work – How to Start Studying

- The more time you put in, the more you will learn. The hardest thing is to start, so let's make it easy for you to get down to work. Just like giving a loading dose of heparin, a boost helps you get started.
  - Make sure your work environment is comfortable, tidy and usable.

- List the tasks you want to complete before you start and make them achievable. Could be 'finish half of the cardiology MKSAP questions by end of today' or 'type up that summary of SLE to explain that silly nephropathy question – finish by lunch'.
- Write down in an obvious place that your goal is to pass the Written Exam. Having this at eye level will give a boost of encouragement when the grey mist of boredom sinks in.

- Study efficiently and effectively in small, regular chunks of time. Make use of the precious spare time you may get during the working day. Instead of spending 30 minutes procrastinating in the RMO room, read that review article with a cup of coffee in your hand.
- Once you've done your chunk of study, tidy up so the space is inviting for next time. File your notes and articles electronically or in folders so you don't waste time hunting during the next session.
- Give yourself a reward for your session. Just like a star chart for a toddler or a doggie treat for a golden retriever, a small reward such as meeting a friend for coffee after three sessions will encourage good behaviour. The size of the reward will depend on your needs and your budget. Make your rewards regular and meaningful.
- Make study fun or at least tolerable. You will know your best time of day. Maybe first thing in the morning, perhaps after dinner. Timetable regular study group sessions each week. Make this realistic and achievable. It is hard to study and work and have a life at the same time.

Here is a timetable from an imaginary registrar who is fairly organised. You'll see that he or she could not study every day, but squeezed in study-chunks throughout the week. It all adds up to a good amount of study fig (f).

(f) **A Weekly Timetable**

Typical week	Monday	Tuesday	Wednesday	Thursday	Friday	Saturday	Sunday
Week 1 What's on	On call, all day and night	Post-take day	Usual day Study group tonight	Football practice	Usual day	Going to movies and football game	Visiting niece in morning
Realistic study sessions	Zero	35 mins before bed	35 mins in morning pre-work	2 × 35 mins after dinner	Zero – rest	3 × 35 mins morning 2 × 35 mins after footie game	4 × 35 mins in afternoon
Week 2 What's on	Post-take day	Usual day	Usual day	Presenting at grand round	Usual day	Drop kids off at grandparents	Son has birthday party
Realistic study sessions	35 mins at work before clinic	1 × 35 mins before work 1 × 35 mins after yoga	Zero – doing grand round slides	Zero	Zero – rest	3 × 35 mins in morning 3 × 35 mins after dinner	1 × 35 min after dinner

Summary

- The key reference to this chapter is *Managing your Mind* by Hope and Butler.
- Divide the tasks in your life into four groups: urgent and important, non-urgent and important, urgent and not important, and not urgent and not important. Maximise and prioritise time spent on non-urgent but important tasks through learning to say no, negotiation, outsourcing and understanding the motivations of other people.
- Prioritising your life and minimising less important stuff is good advice for life, and excellent experience for your long case problem list in the Clinical Exam!
- Know where you are on the performance/stress curve. This year, you will be handling a lot more stress. Look after yourself and have strategies to deal with increasing stress levels, so you stay on the good side of the curve.
- If you feel yourself sliding into fatigue or (worse) burnout, have a break and get some help.
- Study in efficient, bite-sized chunks. Incorporate a method where recent topics are revised regularly, as this makes the most of your memory capabilities.
- Organise your study space.
- Reduce distractions, develop a timetable and learn how to get started for a study session.

4

Topics That Need to Be Covered for the Written Exam

Hopefully, you are now in a zen-like state of mindfulness, understand how to manage your own stress levels, think of your life as a pie chart, have employed a cleaner and have resigned yourself to the fact that this is a marathon, not a sprint. You also have realised that this is one massive beast of an exam that will put you through the wringer for a year. It is now time to actually start studying. What comes next is why, and what ground needs to be covered. We will cover specifically what material to study in Chapter 6.

What is My Goal? Why Am I Putting Myself Through This?

It is crucial to remind yourself of this regularly:

> *My goal is to pass the FRACP Written Exam. Sanity prevails.*

Passing this exam is the only way to advance through physician or paediatric training. Being a consultant is a wonderful career, and it is all worth it (on most days). Studying and passing will involve sacrifice and hard work.

It is crucial to remind yourself of this too:

> *My goal is <u>not</u> to Learn Everything There Is About Internal Medicine, as this is the way to madness. Sanity prevails.*

The curriculum is vast and terrifying. Unlike other colleges, there is no short prescribed reading list of books that exam questions reliably

How to Pass the RACP Written and Clinical Exams: The Insider's Guide,
Second Edition. Zoë Raos and Cheryl Johnson.
© 2017 John Wiley & Sons Ltd. Published 2017 by John Wiley & Sons Ltd.

come from. We have dedicated Chapter 6 to tried and true resources and books that focus your study.

How to Think Like An Examiner for the Written Exam

After we sat this exam, we realised that:

- someone, somewhere has to write the questions. Step into the examiner's shoes
- when studying a topic, ask yourself, 'How could this be turned into an MCQ?'
- not every bit of medical minutiae can be phrased in an MCQ format.

When we first started studying a topic, we wallpapered our minds (see Chapter 6) and plugged gaps in our knowledge. This is important, but what becomes increasingly important as the months go by is the ability to critically appraise this information and see whether you can formulate an MCQ. If you and your study buddies have difficulty, this is probably a subject that doesn't lend itself to a question. There are many topics that just can't be turned into an MCQ. When you have cracked it, you will see the world in shades of MCQs:

> With respect to dinner tonight, what meal balances the **least** amount of calories against the **highest likelihood** of satisfaction?

A Big Mac and fries
B Fish and chips
C Tin of soup with toast
D Meat lovers pizza from Pizza Hutt
E Roast chicken with vegetables

You get the point! This is why we are so pleased that MCQ-based study resources are available for trainees.

Organising Your Study Time – A Plan of Attack

With the mountain of information to get through, a plan and timetable kept us going. Other people had a far more relaxed (some might say less anally retentive) approach, started in one area and went where it lead them. Some study groups divided up the year and allowed about three weeks per 'big' topic and one week per 'little' topic. We timed personal study with what our study group was doing that month. Another really good way to organise your study plan is to align topics with the lecture series (see Chapter 6). Whatever you decide, it is motivating and helpful to have a list of topics that you tick off.

You will have to cover the same ground multiple times. Reading all about glomerulonephritis in May doesn't mean that it will still be there nine months later. Don't be disheartened; the second, third and fourth times you re-memorise the CD markers will get progressively easier, and the 35-minute study sessions we mentioned in Chapter 3 mean you will continually revise material in a time-efficient manner.

The FRACP Curriculum

The curriculum continues to evolve and is currently undergoing another revamp to be available online as a living and breathing document. Whatever its current iteration, it is useful as a checklist to make sure all topics are covered. Online resources for guiding study will be in place on the RACP website in the future.

The College wants your knowledge level to be that of a trainee at the end of basic training and not of a specialist. This does cause your authors (once trainees, now teachers) to chuckle softly, as they recall struggling to answer MCQs in their own particular area of interest at the last teaching session …

Topics to Cover

Adult medicine		Paediatrics and child health	
Cardiology	Infectious diseases	Acute care	Haematology
Clinical epidemiology*	Intensive care	Cardiology	Immunology and allergy
Clinical genetics*	Medical oncology	Clinical pharmacology*	Infectious diseases
Dermatology	Nephrology	Community paediatrics	Neonatology

(Continued)

(Continued)

Adult medicine		Paediatrics and child health	
Endocrinology	Neurology	Dermatology	Nephrology
Gastroenterology	Palliative medicine	Development and behaviour	Neurology
Geriatric medicine	Psychiatry	Epidemiology*	Psychiatry
Haematology	Thoracic medicine	Gastroenterology	Rheumatology
Immunology and allergy	Statistics*	Genetics*	Thoracic medicine
Pharmacology*	Rheumatology	Statistics*	Pharmacology*
		Endocrinology	

* Money for jam topics.

This is a rough guide to the topics you will need to revise. When you go through past papers (Chapters 6 & 7), you will note with a heavy heart that the number of pages dedicated to oncology in Harrison's bears no relationship to the number of oncology exam questions. Some years have eight pharmacology questions and seven endocrinology questions. Another year might have 12 geriatrics, four pharmacology, nine respiratory, 0 dermatology, 0 endocrine, two gastroenterology and three ICU questions. In some years, fringe specialties (like rheumatology, dermatology, geriatric medicine and immunology) had the most questions whilst big bread and butter specialties (cardiology, respiratory) had fewer. Every year the proportions change. There is no magic formula that we've yet unearthed. Dear reader, you'll just have to study everything.

Money for Jam

In the list above, we have asterisked money for jam topics. Looking at the looming list of topics to cover, your eyes may glaze over at the thought of calculating the number needed to treat or a hysteresis loop. You may be tempted to leave these out. Don't. These are key topics that come up each year. If you understand the theory then you can nail the question each and every time, which is more than can be said for memorising the markers for type I and type II autoimmune hepatitis. Statistics, epidemiology, pharmacology and genetics might seem difficult or even boring, but they are very important for passing this exam, and the MCQs get much easier with practice and familiarity. To make money for jam topics even trickier, it can be quite hard to track down resources to help. We outline some excellent resources in Chapter 6. Usefully, all the two-week revision courses are well aware of these topics and cover them thoroughly.

Make sure that by the time you go into the exam (ideally, well before you go on the two-week revision course):

- **Punnet squares and family trees are sorted**: seek help if you don't understand how they work because they often come up in exams
- **sensitivity/specificity epidemiology equations and principles are nailed**: questions always come up and you will kick yourself if you fudge this easy mark
- **make a card with the pharmacology equations**: it's worth spending time to understand the equations because past questions are often repeated
- **understand common blood films and CD markers/translocations**: it seems like the same old clinical scenarios come up year after year so make sure you know these.

Immunology – Special Mention

This topic may surprise you. Despite being a niche subspecialty (how often does a medical registrar call an immunologist about a patient?), every year immunology sends its little tentacles into different specialties and therapeutics, which means more exam questions for you. There is now a well-attended immunology weekend for basic physician trainees (see Chapter 8).

An understanding of all the T-helper cells and their CD markers would have made things a lot easier if we'd gone over this topic early in our preparation. We would strongly recommend you know your CD4 from your CD8. There was an excellent series of review articles from the *New England Journal of Medicine* a number of years ago, which make all things immunological a little bit easier to understand. They have great pictures and explain how all the different parts of the immune system link in together. The basics of immune cells, complement and immunoglobulins hasn't changed much. Make sure that you take the time to go through this and work out what each cell does early in your study.

Visual Material in the Exam

When it comes to visual material that the College can throw at you, the following are fair game:

Plain X-rays	CT scans
MRI scans	ECGs
Radioisotope scans	Respiratory function tests
Sleep studies	Blood films
Bone marrow films	Echocardiograms
Electromyograms	Electroencephalograms
Histology sections	DEXA scans

It is possible to get a specialised textbook for every possible investigation, but this is another way to madness. Instead, get to all the radiology and multidisciplinary meetings you can at your hospital. For example, at our hospital, almost every day a department will have a multidisciplinary radiology, histopathology and clinical meeting. This might be gastroenterology, respiratory, colorectal surgery. There are plate rounds for microbiology, echo sessions in cardiology … see what we mean? If you can get to one or two of these meetings per specialty, you will quickly upskill.

Every day, you will be ordering scans, ECGs and goodness knows what else on your patients. Take a few minutes to really interrogate every investigation your patients have against the report, look at the films and quiz your house officer and medical students. This type of learning will be much more valuable on exam day than trying to memorise another textbook.

Summary

- Your goal is to pass this exam. Your goal is NOT to learn everything there is to know about medicine.
- The FRACP curriculum is in evolution, but is still a good place to tick off topics.
- Have a plan of attack for moving through topics from March to October.
- Know your Money for jam (genetics, epidemiology, pharmacology, statistics) topics backwards, forwards and backwards again.
- Immunology is worth studying early, as it reaches into many other topics.
- Use your time at work to upskill at interpreting radiology, histopathology and other visual material that could be thrown at you on exam day.

5

Study Group

Most registrars know about the awesomeness that is being part of a study group. If you've made the commitment to start studying, then now is the time to round up two or three like-minded colleagues and start a study group. Is a study group compulsory? Of course not! Some people work better alone, and they still pass. And some hospitals have such organised teaching programmes that the main purpose of having a study group (i.e. getting together regularly to moan a lot and thrash out old questions) is achieved. Generally speaking, we have observed that those who fail are more likely to not have had a regular study group. A study group allows you to focus on the curriculum, keeps up momentum, gets everyone in the groove of answering MCQs and ensures all relevant topics are covered.

General Principles That Make Study Groups Effective

Every study group works a little differently. However, over the years, we've observed general principles that mark out successful groups.

- Aiming to meet once a week for at least two hours.
- Food and drink helps. Some of us found a good glass of sauvignon blanc infinitely useful.
- Get the number in the group about right. Most had 3–5 members; any more and it turns into a bunfight, any less and waiting for rota gaps is like waiting for the planets to align. Some registrars formed a Skype study group with one other person to great success, a really

How to Pass the RACP Written and Clinical Exams: The Insider's Guide, Second Edition. Zoë Raos and Cheryl Johnson.
© 2017 John Wiley & Sons Ltd. Published 2017 by John Wiley & Sons Ltd.

good solution if you are studying from a small centre, are a single parent or it is difficult to leave the house in the evenings.

- Form a group with registrars you get on with, or at least respect. Occasionally, there can be a mega-meltdown of epic proportions – personality clashes! A hostile takeover of another registrar! Storming out! Sulking over a particularly thorny question! These occurrences are mercifully uncommon with kind-hearted and compassionate FRACP trainees.
- Most groups with a high pass rate have a plan for the year, such as ploughing through each topic's worth of questions before the two-week revision course and moving on to the next topic, even if the previous topic was incomplete. This maintains momentum and focus. For the highly organised, the study group plan would mirror the general plan of the personal revision plan for the individuals. For the less organised, the study group plan would drag them along through the topics – win win!
- It is amazing how different clinical knowledge can be across three or four registrars. With sharing and co-operation, you will learn much from one another.
- The venue was usually each other's houses. Some groups meet at the library or the hospital – we thought we spent quite enough time at the hospital! Meeting at a pub or restaurant sounds like fun, but may not translate into productive work.
- Try to get your study group to the same two-week revision course. There will be fewer problems scheduling study group sessions as everyone is away at the same time, and there will always be someone to have dinner with.

What Do You Do at Study Group?

This varied a lot, as it should. We would go over and around hot topics and old questions. Ideas would bounce around, with one person on a laptop looking through UpToDate, another person flicking through Harrison's, someone else cooking dinner or ordering pizza, the last person complaining noisily about the complete lack of relevance of the question. There were evenings where we would all admit zero knowledge of pharmacology and spend a couple of hours teaching each other all the equations and making sure we got the questions right.

Other groups would set homework. This could include creating summaries and teaching for the others, or going over five MCQ questions each and teaching the rest of the group with worked answers. Some groups would meet more casually, more to share resources than to go over questions or concerns. A good approach would be to ask a senior registrar with whom you identify how they organised their group.

Once you've got your group together, have a talk about how you want the group to work and be flexible about it. A lot of the benefit from study group was sharing the burden/journey of studying with like-minded people. It certainly kept us (mostly) sane!

Summary

- We observe that trainees in a well-organised study group are more likely to pass than those who go it alone.
- Make a study group with like-minded trainees and meet regularly.
- Work out how your particular study group is going to function and plan your study together for the year. Decide how your group will work, and what you will cover.
- Share knowledge.
- Support each other to get through.

6

Now We Know How to Study, What Stuff Do We Study From?

Wallpapering Your Mind

Wallpapering your mind is a little term that describes a very big task – how to bridge the massive gap between being a registrar and being a registrar who is ready to sit the exam. Some candidates have a photographic memory for all minutiae from medical school and all factoids from ward rounds. Then, there's everyone else who must bash through the basics at least once before being able to really understand old exam questions. Internal medicine is both broad and deep, so maintaining a brisk pace as you put up the wallpaper is essential.

The majority of candidates we knew focused on one major wallpapering resource and left the others as reference guides for individual questions. There has been, thankfully, an increase in the marketplace of MCQ-type resources that have taken over from traditional book-based learning for many candidates.

Once you have wallpapered your mind for several months, the furniture (specific, exam-focused information) needs to move in. Everyone who sits this exam is coming from a different background. Some of you may have cardiology knowledge from your CCU SHO days. You may know all about the investigation of jaundice as your boss is a gastroenterologist. Extra furniture will come from looking at old FRACP questions, and reading and debating around them.

Here we have listed some resources that we found useful and that have worked for candidates over the last couple of years. There are many more again, with online websites written by registrars, for registrars. There is no single resource – oh that there was! The resources at your disposal are numerous yet imperfect when it comes to this exam.

How to Pass the RACP Written and Clinical Exams: The Insider's Guide,
Second Edition. Zoë Raos and Cheryl Johnson.
© 2017 John Wiley & Sons Ltd. Published 2017 by John Wiley & Sons Ltd.

Textbooks give an excellent overview of internal medicine but can fail miserably when drilling down into a tricky MCQ; likewise, a Medline search can generate massive confusion which can only be treated by a large gin and tonic. There are not enough hours in the day to do the lecture series *and* the MKSAPS *and* the MRCP MCQs online *and* read Harrison's *and* go over someone else's stuffy study notes. You'll go mad! And that won't help anybody. Do not buy every single text-book and lecture series – even if you are independently wealthy with endless time on your hands, this strategy will overwhelm and confuse. It is worth spending a week asking around and looking at what is on offer, then picking a strategy and sticking to it. Have a good look at the comprehensive list of resources below. Then, we recommend narrowing the list to the following:

- One lecture series. Either your local one or the FRACP Physician Education Programme (PEP). It is possible to do both, or to bounce between the two depending on your commitments week by week.
- One MCQ-based resource *or* ploughing through one medium-sized textbook if you're an old-fashioned studier.
- An UpToDate subscription for reference.
- A couple of big and small reference texts. For reference. That means referring to.

We will discuss old FRACP questions and how to incorporate them into your study in the following chapter.

Comprehensive List of Resources for Wallpapering Your Mind

Lecture-Based Resources

Regional Teaching

Hopefully, your region will have weekly FRACP Written Exam teaching sessions you can attend in person, via videoconference or the web. One advantage of local teaching is the ability to show MCQs to the lecturer. Most lecturers are keen to have a go, prefacing responses with 'What a controversial topic; either of these two answers is technically correct'. After some head scratching, you'll get an explanation that may save you hours of digging around on Google Scholar.

When at teaching, if practical, we gave our pagers to our trusty house officer. He or she would call or message us on our cellphone for queries and emergencies. This meant that we weren't constantly dashing in and out to answer calls. You may have to intermittently bribe your house officer with chocolate for this strategy to work or give them an early afternoon off once in awhile. If there are not weekly lectures at your centre, or if they are not up to scratch, then subscribe to the Physician Education Programme.

Physician Education Programme Lectures (www.racp.edu.au)

The Victorian and Tasmanian Education Committee (VTEC) has run this series of lectures for many years, now hosted by the official RACP website. The cost is currently A\$392 year – less for early birds – and is a reimbursable expense in some centres; 135 lectures are given over 45 Thursday evenings from 6.30 to 9.30 pm Australian time. You can tune in live or download audio and PDFs of the slides for learning on the go. The current group of registrars found these lectures to be excellent, and you could use these lectures as part of your wallpapering timetable rather than reading. It all depends on your learning style. What's really good about a lecture series is you will be dragged kicking and screaming through the topics, and won't fall into the trap of doing nothing but rheumatology for four months. You may also be lucky and find that a consultant presenting a lecture on a pet topic may also write exam questions.

What registrars say about these lectures: 'PEP lectures were a must. It helps plan your study and pace. Not all lectures are interesting, but at least you know what topics to focus on'.

Paeds Point: Auckland University Lectures (www.fracpteaching.com)

A group of Auckland paediatricians arrange a comprehensive training course through the University of Auckland for the Written Exam. This is funded for Auckland-based registrars and currently costs NZ\$3500 for everyone else – hopefully reimbursed as a cost of training in New Zealand and tax deductible in Australia. Paediatric trainees across Australasia give consistent feedback that this is a great lecture series, worth the cost, and improves your chance of passing. The lectures are held on Thursday afternoons from June to February, with two-hour weekly webcasts that can be seen live or at a time that suits. Also included for your hard-earned dosh are practice MCQs each week, recommended reading and a mock exam in February.

MCQ-Based Resources

If there is one thing that makes studying more straightforward now, it is the availability of resources that are based around MCQs. This makes a big difference, as the candidate gets into the groove of MCQs and can use self-assessment to figure out knowledge holes. Plus, you cotton on to what medical knowledge can be turned into an MCQ and what can't. The disadvantage of MCQ-based resources is the trap of mindlessly answering question after question with no active learning. Avoid this trap. If a question uncovers a great gaping hole in your medical knowledge ('Oh, so hepatitis C has genotypes now?'), then *stop and plug that hole.* Do this by reading a chapter in a textbook, a review article or looking on UpToDate. Write some notes and file them neatly away for future revision.

MKSAP: Medical Knowledge Self-Assessment Program Questions

This is a comprehensive MCQ-based resource available as books or e-books, from the American College of Physicians. It is updated every two years and is aimed at US trainees sitting their Board exams and physicians who want to get CME points. Each subject starts with a focus on hot topics in each specialty, followed by MCQs in a 'best answer' format. A full subscription includes 11 books, CD-ROMs and an app for your Apple or Android device. Some centres use MKSAP as a group-teaching tool for their registrars.

As MKSAPs are American, there is a different focus from Australasia and another set of reference ranges to get your head around (there is a table in the back of Harrison's that comes in handy for this). It does miss out money for jam topics such as statistics and pharmacology and is limited in geriatric medicine. The MCQs aren't up to the FRACP levels of eye-watering detail. MKSAPs are an up-to-date way to wallpaper your mind and cover a lot of ground in a time-efficient way. The notes are concise and relevant, the questions get you into 'MCQ mode' and the answers include full explanations. Each chapter/topic takes about 1–2 weeks to go over.

BMJ OnExamination (www.onexamination.com)

The BMJ OnExamination website prepares UK candidates for their MRCP examinations, like MKSAPS for Brits. It is an MCQ-based question bank which is excellent for learning and wallpapering the mind. The questions are kept up to date, so new therapeutics, the latest literature and hot topics are well covered. Explanations are well laid out and logical, but can be brief (UpToDate comes in handy to fill in gaps). Most candidates in our regional hospitals subscribed to OnExamination and liked it. These MCQs are just easy enough to plough through when you're home late or on night duty. They are *not* hard enough to replace old FRACP exam questions. Some candidates used OnExamination as their main wallpapering and would set a goal, such as 10–40 questions per night. There are two parts (1 and 2) that are aligned to the different UK exams. Some trainees chose to cover one part or the other – there is a lot of overlap and simply so many questions it is difficult to get through them all anyway.

Pastest (www.pastest.co.uk)

This is another online paid-subscription MRCP-based MCQ bank. Each question has a difficulty level, so the harder questions are more on a par with the trickiness of FRACP questions. Unfortunately, you can't access the information offline which makes it slightly less user friendly.

Passmedicine (www.passmedicine.com)

Yet another online subscription MRCP-based MCQ bank. Have a look at all of them and work out which one will be best for you.

Paeds Point

BMJ OnExamination has about 2000 MCQ-type resources in the MRCPCH section. Each section is tailored to a different part of their curriculum, for example, the Part 1 paeds exams and the paeds diploma. The Brits examine their paeds trainees not just with 'best of 5' MCQs, but with short answer questions and other assessments which are less useful for those studying for the FRACP Written Exam. We have not yet received any reviews from paediatric registrars who have used OnExamination, but given how useful the adult medicine trainees find it, we would suggest it is worth subscribing for a month or two to go over the 'best of 5' MCQs in OnExamination and see what you think. The Part 1 and 2 questions seem more aligned to the FRACP level of difficulty than the diploma questions.

This little book is aimed at North Americans sitting their Board exams. It is divided into sections by topic. A lot of our generation bought this book and raved about it. With the advent of online MCQ resources, fewer trainees use it. Like OnExamination and MKSAP, the questions are in a different style from College MCQs, so this book is no substitute for old questions. It is a nice manageable size, is divided into sections and is a great book to have on hand for rainy afternoons when your broadband connection has crashed and nothing else seems remotely palatable.

Textbooks and Online Resources

There has been a swing away from candidates relying purely on textbooks to prepare for the exam. Nonetheless, we recommend having one or two of the following available for money for jam, wallpapering and digging out answers to sticky questions. Borrow a few books from your local hospital library, university library or a colleague and then choose what suits.

UpToDate (UTD)

In our region, there is universal use of this excellent computer-based resource for all trainees studying for the FRACP Written Exam. Your hospital may have a site licence that allows anybody access to UTD from that workplace. If you need to pay for it, UTD is worth the money. This is a reimbursable expense for many NZ candidates, and is tax deductible for Aussies.

Once the UTD people have beaten up your credit card, you can download it to your mobile device and computer with login-password web-based access. As a 'trainee', you can currently get an annual subscription for around US$200 with an extra US$50 for a mobile app (which also makes you appear clever for ward rounds).

You must dip in and out of UTD and not get bogged down by the wealth of information. It can suck you in with incredible detail for some topics so use it wisely and critically. Like many good things in life, you need to know when to stop.

We used UTD every time we studied, and candidates still rave about it. UTD is the best resource for quickly getting answers to specific questions. There are excellent pictures and radiology, it's searchable, and the summaries of relevant articles contain explanations of the evidence at hand. You can find excellent management strategies that you can't find in the textbooks and of course… it's UpToDate. There is a 'what's new' section with summaries of recent trials separated by topic.

Current Medical Diagnosis and Treatment (Papadakis and McPhee)

CMDT is an annually updated textbook about the size of a phone book, put out by Lange. Quite a few of us old codgers used CMDT; with the advent of MCQ-based resources, it has a place but is not as popular. The text is pithy, easy to understand, well set out, clinically relevant and updated annually. We read CMDT and understood it the first time. There are tables and summaries that are easy to memorise, and the latest edition (electronic and paper) includes illustrations and radiology (not as many as other resources, but a welcome improvement). Clinically focused, CMDT lacks the background science sometimes needed for the medical sciences paper. It is well indexed with good references. It gives you a solid foundation from which to start when you are tackling a subject and you can add detail with Harrison's or UpToDate. Good wallpapering fodder, and exam questions can sometimes be answered. Available on Kindle and there is an app for iPhone and iPad.

Harrison's Principles of Internal Medicine, 19th edition (Kasper and Fauci)

This stalwart of a textbook is what your more ancient consultants may have used as a sole resource. They may freak you out by saying 'I read Harry's twice before the Dunedin Course. What page are you up to?'. They may not be aware that Harry's is now a double-volume behemoth printed on tissue paper complete with a website, a blog and its own gravitational field. Reading it cover to cover is not recommended for modern candidates.

The 19th edition continues to build on improving layout, with lovely diagrams, blood films, radiology and summary tables. Harry's is available as an e-book with a supporting website (www.harrisonsim.com) available if you buy the book. Basic science (genetics, cardiac physiology, oncology, the cell cycle, etc.) is well covered, and saves you wading through physiology or organic chemistry texts.

The writing style and small font are challenging to the tired eyes and brain of a busy medical registrar. Hot topics get out of date in the paper version. The page you look up in the index is always in the other volume. These weaknesses are overcome by using the searchable online version.

Harrison's is an excellent reference text and can be a great help in finding the answers for past exam questions, especially in the medical sciences paper, and useful for settling arguments at study group.

Oxford Textbook of Medicine, 5th edition (Warrell and Cox)
This behemoth has a BMI of 60+. A few people find this to be an excellent reference (we haven't met any of these people because they are off work with back injuries). While the contents are well written and finely detailed, the Oxford is big. And it costs $1000.

Paeds Point

***Nelson Textbook of Pediatrics*, 20th edition (Kliegman and Stanton)**
This is the definitive textbook of paediatrics, and most trainees have a copy that is well thumbed through. After the Written Exam, it is commonly found as a door-stop or being used to prop up a table leg. We have not heard of anyone who read it cover to cover; rather, it is used as a reference for specific questions. There is an e-book version and a supporting website.

***Concise Paediatrics*, 2nd edition (Sidwell and Thomson)**
This is a far leaner book than Nelson and is commonly used for paediatric mind wallpapering to ensure all topics are covered. It is aimed at UK paediatric trainees. Much like CMDT, it does not contain the level of detail required to answer the more esoteric FRACP questions, but nonetheless is a well-liked text that will take you through the big and small topics. Buy it.

UpToDate
This is an excellent online resource for paeds candidates too. Subscribe.

Other Useful Textbooks and Resources

Passing the FRACP Written Examination – Questions and Answers
(Gleadle et al.)
This quality small book is written specifically about the adult medicine FRACP exam. It contains MCQs and a good choice of hot topics in certain areas. Everyone found the layout to be difficult to navigate

as the questions and answers are in different areas, and require you to flick back and forth. This minor annoyance aside, the questions are up to FRACP standard, the explanations and answers were indepth and the list of recommended journal articles is comprehensive. Like all printed material, the content will date in fast-moving specialties, so let's hope the authors continue to keep this handy book up to date with further publications. It is not comprehensive enough to be a sole MCQ resource for wallpapering, but is worth your consideration.

Internal Medicine: The Essential Facts, 3rd edition (Talley et al.)
This book is a gem. The 2014 edition has been revised and is bigger and brighter than the 1999 antique we relied on to tackle money for jam questions. Money well spent, full of clinical pearls, helpful tables and pretty diagrams that make pharmacology almost understandable. It contains chapters on finicky topics that historically generate loads of questions, like pharmacology, genetics and statistics.

First Aid for the USMLE Step 1 (Le and Bhushan)
This little American gem is fantastic for medical sciences and money for jam questions. Contains lots of concise summaries along with nice pictures, good mnemonics and simple explanations. There are some sections that are not relevant for an Australasian exam. The book is updated yearly.

Pharmacokinetics Made Easy (Convenors of the Dunedin MCQ course)
This little book, handed out to those who attend the Dunedin MCQ course (see Chapter 8), is gold for all your clinical pharmacology learning. It covers everything from clearance, volume of distribution and half-life to therapeutic drug monitoring and has MCQs to consolidate your learning. As the pages progress, the material gets less relevant and more difficult to understand, so let exam questions be your guide. May be difficult to come by, so ask colleagues who have recently finished the exam for a copy.

Clinical Examination: A Systematic Guide to Physical Diagnosis, 7th edition (Talley and O'Connor)
Examination Medicine: A Guide to Physician Training, 6th edition (Talley and O'Connor)
These two clinical medicine books are essential for the Clinical Exam but are totally worth a read through now. There is an excellent chapter

in the *Examination Medicine* book about preparing for the Written Exam. See Chapter 13 for full reviews of these books.

Course Notes

Course notes from a previous Melbourne, Dunedin or Sydney course give you a good idea of where to start, hot topics and the level required to answer real-life FRACP questions. Money for jam topics are almost always well covered. The topics covered are not exhaustive, so we do not suggest using these as a sole wallpapering resource. While these notes are great, they are no replacement for attending a course. See Chapter 8 and book yourself into a course now.

Other Handy Resources for Wallpapering and MCQ Sleuthing
- Good ol' little Oxford yellow handbook
- Your local clinical handbooks
- Your local hospital intranet, e.g. antimicrobial guidelines

Technological Advances to Help With Your Study

Dropbox
Technology has advanced significantly from when we sat the exam and passed corruptible USB memory sticks around. Cloud-based computing has revolutionised the sharing and storing of information and saved a few trees. Dropbox is good for two purposes: first, you can access your own notes wherever you are, and second, you can share information amongst your study group or more widely amongst the trainees in your hospital. Sharing is caring, people...

WhatsApp/Other Large Group Forums
WhatsApp is a cross-platform mobile messaging application that allows multiple users to exchange messages without paying for texts. You can create a forum of 20+ people, post those difficult MCQs and then discuss possible answers. Facebook is another alternative and previous registrars have posted MCQs to get responses from other currently studying registrars or those who have passed the exams. You are only limited by your friend base!

There are multiple large group platforms for sharing information, discussing tricky medical problems and networking. Some current ones include Doximity, OPENPaediatrics and FOAMed and no doubt there will be more on the scene over time. We don't know anyone who has used them to help with their study but we welcome any recommendations or reviews. It may be worth spending a short time looking at them and seeing whether they may work for you and your study buddies.

Be judicious – too much time in these fora can quickly suck you into the 'not urgent and not important' slice of the pie chart (see Chapter 3).

Journals: A Suggested Approach

Many candidates claim that they never read a journal article and still passed. Others read too many randomly, wasted time and burnt out. We have noticed that more questions are coming straight out of journals as the College keeps topics up to the minute and reduces the number of repeated questions. Thankfully, the conveners of hospital lecture series and two-week exam courses will do some of the hard work for you. The only slightly comforting thought is that the exam questions are written, locked down and loaded by the preceding October.

There are seven journals that the College recommends you read. That is a lot, too many really, and to follow all seven would take too much time away from wallpapering and getting used to MCQs. Of late, the 'Big Three' of *Internal Medicine Journal*, *Lancet* and *New England Journal of Medicine* have been good hunting grounds for possible questions.

What most trainees do, and what we did, was focus on review articles from the Big Three. If a question is going to be written from a journal, usually it will be uplifted from a review article unless it is a great big game-changing trial. Ask your consultants and senior registrars about game-changing papers. Attending and presenting at your local journal club is a time-efficient way of doing this.

Review articles are an excellent way to fill in a knowledge deficit. For example, autoimmune hepatitis or sarcoid may have always eluded you. Reading a good review article is a time-efficient way to plug that gap. But don't get too bogged down in the minutiae of review articles, particularly if they are super-specialised.

Paeds Point
The journal that has the highest chance of containing review articles that generate questions is the good old RACP stalwart *Paediatrics and Child Health*. Other medium-sized hitters are *Archives of Disease in Childhood*, *Pediatric Clinics of North America* and *Pediatrics*. If a really big paediatric trial or review article appears in the *Lancet*, *BMJ* or *NEJM* then take note, an exam question could easily come from there too.

Useful Websites

www.racp.edu.au
This is the official College website. There are all sorts of resources, the training portal, sample questions and information about how the examination is scaled. You can also access the *Internal Medicine Journal*. As we will discuss in Chapter 7, you can no longer download old RACP Written Exam papers from the website.

www.passthefracp.com
This unofficial Australian website has remembered questions, resources and lecture notes. Well worth a look around.

www.tga.gov.au
The ADRAC website is useful for pharmacology questions. If you click on 'recalls and alerts', the ADRAC stuff is under the 'alerts' heading.

www.medsafe.govt.nz
Medsafe writes individual drug summaries for all prescribed medications in New Zealand. The datasheets are to the point yet comprehensive – this will save you time. There is a 'hot topics' section with alerts on important drug interactions.

www.medlib.med.utah.edu
This site is good for renal biopsy and haematology slide sections. MCQs are included which are good if you're on nights or in a study funk.

www.labplus.co.nz
This big Auckland lab has a website that is dated and clunky, but clicking through 'Clinical Resources' to 'Test Guide' reveals gold for interpreting lab test results. Current registrars found the endocrinology test summaries to be particularly useful.

www.dermnetnz.org
This is an excellent website for all things dermatological. Includes clinical summaries and photographs, and covers skin manifestations of other conditions. Well worth adding to your bookmark page, and excellent for answering most exam questions where a rash is involved.

www.wellingtonicu.com/Education/Resources/Tripp/

David Tripp is an ICU consultant in Wellington. Having sat the FRACP exam a few years ago, he wrote notes for each topic then updated them, most recently in 2009. They are free for all and succinct. David is clearly an over-achiever, as he also has notes for the ICU finals, medical school and the paeds diploma. Double-check the information presented is up to date.

Summary

- Wallpapering your mind creates a solid foundation for each topic, with detail added on top. Most candidates wallpaper by themselves with individual study, and add detail with past FRACP questions through study group sessions and attending lectures.
- There are loads of resources available. Choose which one to focus on according to your learning style. Most candidates pick one MCQ-based resource and one big textbook, subscribe to UpToDate and invest in one or two smaller books to cover money for jam topics.
- MCQ resources are fantastic but make your learning active. If you identify a gap in your knowledge in an MCQ, stop and bridge that gap with focused study.
- Questions can come straight out of certain journal articles; be judicious as reading too many journals can bog you down.

7

Old FRACP Exam Questions

In the old days, most of us studied like this.

- We wallpapered our minds by studying each topic in the FRACP curriculum, aiming to get through everything once by November.
- We tackled old FRACP MCQs in our study group (back then old papers were easily available from the College), as well as revising hot topics from recent years where papers weren't published. Every single old hand who had passed the exam would impress upon us that the key to passing was to do old papers and hot topics. We did – it worked.
- We went along to a two-week revision course, got scared and a big kick up the proverbial.
- Boned up on hot topics and money for jam.
- Post course, all study efforts were ramped up. More old questions done under exam conditions
- Exam day.

We knew excellent candidates who studied hard, but did not base their study around the FRACP questions, and failed. We knew candidates who based all their study only around old exam questions and did no wallpapering, and failed. The key for us – a mixture of both.

Old FRACP papers were an absolutely crucial part of our revision for the exam. We used old questions as a way of focusing our study on important topics, finding a review article on a particular disease and getting to grips with the level of detail required.

As the Written Exam drew closer, we did old exams all over again 'under exam conditions'. This was useful to practise exam time management, and gave us an accurate picture of our progress.

How to Pass the RACP Written and Clinical Exams: The Insider's Guide, Second Edition. Zoë Raos and Cheryl Johnson.
© 2017 John Wiley & Sons Ltd. Published 2017 by John Wiley & Sons Ltd.

There has been a big change in recent years because the College wants to create a great big question bank so that more discriminating questions are available to the examiners when/if there is a move to a biannual exam. *The College has now taken all past papers off the website.* All that remains is a skerrick of sample questions, leaving a great big hole in what was a crucial part of revision.

As for hot topics, the College frowns heavily upon those who sit down at the end of the exam, write down all that they can remember, type it all up and pass it on as this means questions are less able to discriminate amongst candidates. You will be asked to sign a 'waiver' prior to the exam that states you will not copy or recreate the exam questions.

Without Us, or You, Breaking the Rules, How Can the Modern Candidate Cope Without FRACP Past and Remembered Papers?

Past exam sitters and certain websites will have old exam papers on a cloud or hard drive. Get networking and find whatever you can. Even if the questions are five or 10 years old, you will get a feel for the style of questions to expect on exam day, and how to answer them. We also think it is not unreasonable to ask those who have just sat, in general terms, about topics that came up in their exam without compromising anybody. In the two-week courses, hot topics from the last few years are well covered. Also, every revision course has a mock exam, so track down mock exam MCQs from courses for the past few years and you will have some nice sticky questions and hot topics to work with over your year of study. And at least these days there are UK MCQ resources to study from (see Chapter 6).

What is the Point of Doing Old FRACP and Course Questions?

Old questions may as well be written in ancient Greek when you first start doing them. The language of FRACP questions becomes more familiar with time, which is why we found it crucial to get stuck in early. By doing old papers, you are continuously assessing yourself, familiarising yourself with the way the examiners think and understanding the depth of detail needed to pass a question. There is no point in saving old papers to go over the month before the exam. We integrated old questions into our study programme, especially at study group.

There aren't as many repeated questions as there have been in past years, but the College does repeat a few questions every year (with variations in wording and scenarios). When you're in the Written Exam, those repeated questions are old friends. Even if they are poor discriminators and count less towards your final grade, they buoy confidence on the day and a correct answer is always a win.

Beware – older papers have questions that can be so out of date that the answers are wrong. Even so, go through them with a grain of salt. We rewrote out-of-date questions which was a useful exercise in itself and prompts you to read around the topic.

Someone from each revision course should bring back an unmarked copy of their mock exam to share with colleagues who went to another course. This way, you and your friends will get another 'bank' of questions to practise and use as revision for the final lead-in to exam day.

The key to studying from an MCQ is not only to come up with the right answer, but *why* it is the right response, why the other responses are wrong and to know that topic inside out. While questions are not often repeated, themes and topics flow from year to year which is why it is so tough that old papers are no longer published. Carefully revise these themes. See Chapter 9 for more tips on answering MCQs under exam conditions.

Summary

- The College has very recently removed all old papers from the website.
- Track down whatever old FRACP questions, exams and mock exams that you can.
- Use these questions from early on in your study, in parallel to wallpapering your mind.
- Getting the answer right is only 10% of the work needed for you to pass on exam day. You need to know the theme and topic of that question inside and out.
- There are fewer repeated questions now than there used to be, but themes and hot topics still run from year to year.
- It is essential as the exam draws ever closer to do MCQs under exam conditions, so you can work under time pressure.

8

Two-Week Revision Courses

These excellent and oversubscribed courses are held about four months out from the exam. The dates vary slightly year by year. You must organise your place on a course 6–9 months before, at least. Each course aims to cover new and important areas of the syllabus and includes a mock exam. They all cover hot topics, all cost about the same and are all of an excellent standard. You only need to go to one course.

These courses are great, *if* you have done the work leading up to them by wallpapering and going through questions. These days, it is not at all advisable to start studying from November, there just isn't time to get through all the pesky-mabs, CD4 cells and Punnet squares.

We suggest trying to get to the same course as at least one other person from your study group, ideally all of you. Organise somewhere decent and nearby to stay while you are there. The course fees, airfares and accommodation will be refunded for Kiwis under the current contract (but car hire, nights on the tiles and prime seats at *Phantom of the Opera* are not). If you are Australian, the current $2000 course fee is money well spent, and tax deductible.

Hopefully you'll have fun and learn a great deal. Most of us found the experience of lectures without interruptions from our job and other commitments to be quite mind-blowing (med school is wasted on students!). On the first night, we tried to revise what we learned that day. We gave up on the second night. It was just too intense to sit in lectures all day then try and study, and much more fruitful to go for a walk and find somewhere nice for dinner.

How to Pass the RACP Written and Clinical Exams: The Insider's Guide, Second Edition. Zoë Raos and Cheryl Johnson.
© 2017 John Wiley & Sons Ltd. Published 2017 by John Wiley & Sons Ltd.

You'll go home with about 8 kilograms of notes so pack light. If your course was scanty in a particular area, you can go through someone's material from another course to fill in the gaps once you're home.

There are specialised, shorter revision courses – great if you've got the time and money, but are not as essential.

Whichever course you go to, make sure you sit the mock exam and take a copy home to share.

Sometimes mock questions are clunky, but the topic is the key point. During the mock exam, practise skills like keeping to time and avoiding 'frame shift' errors. You will learn more from failure – this will focus your awareness on areas of weakness. Many candidates have scored 15% in the mocks, cried, got their act together and gone on to pass the actual exam.

Dunedin FRACP Written Examination Revision Course

Contact:
Linda Cunningham
Department of Medicine, Dunedin School of Medicine
University of Otago, PO Box 56, Dunedin 9054
New Zealand
Telephone: (+64 3) 474 0999 ext 8520
Fax: (+64 3) 470 9916
Email: linda.cunningham@otago.ac.nz
Web: www.otago.ac.nz – register online

This excellent 11-day residential course starts with revision in specialty areas, covers hot topics (including pharmacology, thank goodness) and ends with a mock exam (including a really useful session where answers are discussed). There are friendly local, national and international lecturers of considerable repute. You will get a big pile of resource material and notes to take home.

Dunedin is a lovely university town in New Zealand's South Island. There is good food and a range of accommodation options and it is a short drive to many beautiful sights (if you can spare the time). Dress warmly and bring along a smart outfit for the dinner dance at Larnach Castle.

FRACP Written Exam Prep Course – Melbourne

Contact:
DeltaMed
53/135 Cardigan Street, Carlton, VIC 3053
Australia
Telephone: (+61 3) 9347 2718
Fax: (+61 3) 9347 2918
Email: info@deltamed.com.au
Website: www.deltamed.com.au – register online

This course is excellent. Attendees appreciate the memory-friendly time-table of two lectures then a break. There is a mock exam; recent candidates commented that there is not much time to revise the answers during the course itself, but doing this when back home for study group is a good exercise anyway. The study notes are quality but bulky – pack light so there is room in your luggage allowance for the return journey home.

Melbourne is a cosmopolitan city with fantastic food, shopping and culture. You will be kept busy by the lectures, but any free time will be thoroughly enjoyed.

Royal Prince Alfred BPT Exam Revision Course – Sydney

Contact:
Sue Alexander
Clinical Training Unit
Royal Prince Alfred Hospital, Missenden Road, Camperdown, NSW 2050
Australia
Telephone: (+61 2) 9515 6306
Fax: (+61 3) 9515 8173
Email: sue.alexander@sswahs.nsw.govt.au
Web: www.sswahs.nsw.gov.au/rpa/BPTCourse

This excellent 10-day course covers all examinable specialty areas and hot topics. Speakers are local and regional experts, and they use an audience response system to help the more shy attendees participate in discussion.

Sydney is a beautiful city. In November, it might be just warm enough to have a swim at the beach. The venue is a short distance on public transport to the city. The food and shopping are excellent.

Paeds Point

Residential Course in Paediatrics for Part 1 FRACP

Contact:
FRACP Course Administration
Department of Paediatrics
The University of Auckland
Private Bag 92019
Auckland, 1142
fracpadmin@auckland.ac.nz

This full-time two-week residential course complements the year-long lecture series through the University of Auckland. Places are strictly limited to about 50 participants, locals get first dibs and it is always oversubscribed. It is an excellent course by all accounts.

Aljesal FRACP Preparation Course – Sydney

Contact:
kathrynthacker@aljesal.com.au
+61 2 9716 8889

Our paediatric contributors are Auckland trained, so we have not received a first-hand review about the Aljesal course held in Sydney each September. It is a 10-day course, has run for 18 years, is attended by around 100 candidates per year and has a really good reputation. Topics covered are exam focused and there is a mock exam.

Short Courses Worthy of Consideration

DeltaMed MCQ Weekend Courses – Sydney and Melbourne

These are two-day 'last minute revision' courses in Australia that run a month before the Written Exam. They are identical presentations in two different cities (Melbourne and Sydney). They are not a replacement for the two-week courses. About an hour is spent on each topic, with a heavy focus on hot topics. There is an excellent mock exam. The cost is currently around A$363 + travel + accommodation.

DeltaMed Medical Investigations – Melbourne

This one-dayer is held midway through the year and is aimed at trainees who want an exam-focused understanding of medical investigations. We've received mixed reviews but those who struggle to interpret results may find this a useful adjunct.

Contact for DeltaMed courses:
DeltaMed
53/135 Cardigan Street, Carlton, VIC 3053
Australia
Telephone: (+61 3) 9347 2718
Fax: (+61 3) 9347 2918
Email: info@deltamed.com.au
Website: www.deltamed.com.au – register online

Immunology4BPTs

This weekend course in November is run out of Westmead in Sydney. It is designed to demystify immunology so that candidates can nail basic science and clinical immunological questions. It is relevant to adult and paediatric trainees. If this is a real area of weakness, this could be a good course for you. Some individuals found this to be excellent, others thought it too complex and others too simple! We suggest making up your own mind by talking to someone who has gone and looking at the programme on the website.

Contact:
Web: www.immunology4bpts.com

Genetics for Trainees

This is a Melbourne-based course to make genetics (money for jam) understandable. The course is one day long for adult med trainees and two days for paeds. Both lots of trainees attend day 1, including a mock exam based around the adult exam. Day two is just for the paeds cohort with a bigger focus on dysmorphology, with a paeds mock exam at the end. We have not received first-hand feedback from our sources, but the website has good sample questions for everyone and places on the course fill fast. If you like the sound of this course, register your interest early and ask for recommendations from your local trainees.

Contact:
Web: www.geneticsfortrainees.com.au
Email: info@geneticsfortrainees.com.au

Summary

- The two-week revision courses are absolutely excellent. You can't go wrong with any of them. Go, enjoy yourself and make the most of your time to learn and relax.
- Book your two-week course early, confirm your place by paying and make sure you have leave. Have a back-up plan in case your first preference of course is booked.
- Sit the mock exam, even if you are nervous and fear failure.
- Shorter courses held throughout the year are useful but not essential – have a chat to those who have recently done the exam to get their feedback before you commit.
- New revision courses will come on the market as demand increases. Keep your ear to the ground and ask around.

9

Putting It All Together – The Final Three Months

After your two-week course, you will have three months to pull it all together. This final stagger to the finish line is really important. Momentum must be maintained and built upon. Increasing amounts of time and energy will be spent on revision. Study group really comes into its own – we met more often to go over questions and keep each other sane.

Practicalities of Getting to the Exam

Make sure you've received all the official paperwork from the College needed for sitting on the day. Arrange any travel or accommodation for the exam well in advance. If your exam is not in your hometown, then plan one or two days in advance to recover from the journey and allow for delays.

What to Study

In these last 12 weeks, most candidates revise the material from the course, and if a section was sub par, look at sections from friends who went to other courses. Exam questions are incredibly important now. Make sure you are practising old exams and mock exams under proper, timed, examination conditions.

Many of us had a notebook or file entitled 'stuff that I have to memorise the day before the exam'. We all have little memory holes – this is a nice way of keeping them in check.

How to Pass the RACP Written and Clinical Exams: The Insider's Guide,
Second Edition. Zoë Raos and Cheryl Johnson.
© 2017 John Wiley & Sons Ltd. Published 2017 by John Wiley & Sons Ltd.

Keeping as Calm as Possible

With increasing pressure comes increasing stress, so plot your position on the stress–performance curve (Chapter 3). Look after yourself, keep calm and keep positive. This is far easier said than done. I still remember with the utmost clarity when my now-husband came home to find me sitting on the sofa, in the dark, sobbing, surrounded by piles of memory cards.

> BEN: Are you paralysed by fear again?
> ME: Yip.
> BEN: Cup of tea, wine or box of tissues?
> ME: Wine. And tissues. Then tea. Thank you.

It really was awful at times, but we got through. We couldn't have done it without family and the friends we studied with. Stick together, and contain the self-doubt so it does not take up any more time than it has to.

Leading Up to the Big Day – The Weeks Before

- **Work:** plan your shifts well ahead with leave days and swaps to stay on the straight and narrow. Talk with your Director of Physician Training if there are problems.
- **Home:** eat good-quality food. Keep exercising. Get to bed early. Practise good sleep hygiene. Hopefully, the people around you are used to all the study and stress, will be glad when it's over and are providing support and sustenance.
- **Self-management:** pre-exam nerves are normal. It is normal to worry and be anxious. It is also normal to have exaggerated and unrealistic negative expectations – 'I am sure to fail'. These kinds of thoughts can become increasingly intrusive as the exam draws closer. You may also catastrophise that your entire life will go to pot as well – 'I am a terrible registrar', 'My boyfriend hates me', 'I am the worst goalie in the history of hockey' or 'I will never be able to knit again'. Hopefully, these thoughts will ease off after the exam. Try and ignore them by distraction and focusing on your preparation. Relaxation techniques (meditation, mindfulness and progressive muscle relaxation) are helpful for many.

- **Revision:** if nothing else, study itself can help ease your nerves. Focus on hot topics, themes from old questions and money for jam topics. Don't waste your time revising topics that it would be hard to write a question about. Only look at old questions and your condensed notes. Brand new material, unless of crucial importance, could freak you out.
- **Mind games:** use them. If you've followed our advice, you have spent close to a year preparing for this exam. You attended a two-week course, have gone over and over your summaries and have spent countless hours thrashing out exam questions at study group. The key thing now is to remain calm and keep your eye on the prize.
- **Plan your timing:** get ready for exam day by doing questions and papers under exam conditions. Practise sticking to 1.6 minutes per question. Some questions take 20 seconds to answer, others four minutes so it is crucial in these final few weeks to decide on your timing on the day and get used to it. Make sure any travel to the exam is checked and confirmed.
- **Other candidates:** be supportive of your study buddies. Look out for the stress monkeys – anxiety is contagious. Offer general support but avoid getting trapped in someone else's freak-out-a-thon. If you detect an imminent meltdown in the ranks, enlist immediate and effective support from people who are *not* sitting the exam so that those who are (including you, dear reader) do not unravel in tandem.

The Day Before

Make sure you know where to go and where to park. Some folk swear by a 'rehearsal' – looking around the exam centre the day before to increase familiarity with the surroundings.

Buy spare pencils and erasers, a sippy bottle of water and some non-noisy nutritious snacks for the day. Get all the paperwork from the College together. Get some rest. If you've made a little notebook called 'stuff to go over the day before the exam' then now is the time to read it. Spend a couple of hours, but no more, on last minute pesky-mabs, tumor markers, pharmacology equations and Punnet squares – all those things that need to be memorised.

Go to bed early and get a good night's sleep – that alone is worth at least 10 marks.

On the Day – How to Get Through the Exam

Morning
Paper 1 – Medical Sciences: 70 questions; time allowed: 2 hours
Lunch break (where no one really eats that much)
Afternoon
Paper 2 – Clinical Applications: 100 questions; time allowed: 3 hours

Make sure you are rested, fed and watered on the morning and wearing comfortable clothes and shoes. Have a healthy breakfast and make your daily dose of caffeine on the lower side of normal; your adrenal glands will take care of the rest. Put on your watch, otherwise (like Cheryl) you will be scrambling around on the day borrowing someone else's.

If you're sitting in the city you live in, you might be a nervous wreck on the roads (literally). Best not to drive. Ask someone to drop you off, take the train or share a taxi with a kindred spirit to Exam Central. Arrive for your exam with plenty of time. If you get there early, chill out and watch the world go by on a park bench or find a nice café nearby.

Avoid stress monkeys like the plague or you might bite off your last remaining fingernail. Remember – anxiety is contagious. If you detect a major wobble from another candidate, do not get overly involved. Offer brief support, then immediately outsource the role of support person to College staff or people who are *not* sitting the exam today. Your job today is to sit the exam and do your best.

Make your way to the exam centre well before time. The invigilators will invite you into the room. Make sure you've got everything you need, and all contraband (electronic devices, notes) is left outside the room.

So now you're sitting in the room. Calm your jangled nerves. Breathe.

- Read all the instructions on the front of the paper.
- In the few minutes before the clock starts, plan your attack. Time management is crucial. Allow about 1.6 minutes per question. Many excellent candidates have failed because they couldn't get through the questions. Write down your timing – 'finish 35 questions in the first hour'.

- The invigilators will start the clock. Open the paper.
- For each question, read the stem carefully. Carefully underline key words (e.g. 'works as <u>oyster</u> farmer' and '<u>least</u> likely'). Remember that 'the best investigation', 'the next investigation' and 'the most appropriate investigation' can all be very different things.
- For standard MCQs, go through each of the possible answers and cross them off if they are wrong. Remember, they're not called distracters for nothing! Most of the time, this method will get it down to two possible answers.
- When faced with two possible answers, think back to patients you have seen in the past and remember what management option you took – if in doubt, think 'What would my boss do?' as your consultants are usually right!
- As you shade in each response, double-check that you are answering the right question.
- Some of the questions in the exam will have an obvious correct answer, some can be whittled down to a couple of options and others will be a guess. The main thing is to make it as intelligent a guess as possible.
- Make your first attempt at a question your best but mark the question paper if you think you need to come back and try again. Leaving a square blank is risky, as you might do a massive frameshift error or forget to come back. You need a clear system of identifying what questions you want to return to for a second look if time allows.
- If you are stuck, go back to the stem and ask yourself 'What point are they making?'. The examiners are not trying to trick you. They are usually making an important point about some aspect of diagnosis or management. If your mind remains blank, scribble notes about the topic in the margin. Sometimes this jogs the memory into action, perhaps enough to at least rule out one crazy response. If you really are stuck, pick a letter at random and *move on* to the next question. Your subconscious will continue to mull over the question and hopefully you will get a Eureka moment later on. Moving on is absolutely key in this exam. Candidates have failed by spending far too long on tricky questions.
- Many candidates will tell you never to change your first answer. This is especially true if you're not sure of an answer; your gut reaction is probably right. However, if you've made a blindingly obvious mistake (e.g. thought it was 'most likely' when it was 'least likely' or you miscalculated a maths question) then change it. One candidate reckons she changed about 10 of her answers and she got through.

- Regularly check that you have not made a frameshift error with your answers. You don't want to discover this fatal mistake at the end of the exam.

Summary

- As many a wise parent has said, 'get your ducks in a row' before the exam – preparation is key in the final countdown. This includes keeping sane, rested and in control as much as possible for those last few months. Be organised and use study leave and swaps so that back-to-back shifts and night duties are minimised.
- After your two-week course, revise the notes. Do the mock exam, and MCQs from other two-week courses, under exam conditions (even if you have looked at those questions before). Do old FRACP questions also under exam conditions.
- Organise travel to the exam centre to allow for any delays.
- Three months out, start a file or notebook called 'the day before the exam – stuff I want to look at'. This might include pharmacology equations, a hot topic that came up in the course or facts you always forget.
- In the final few weeks, look after yourself and manage the stress levels as best you can. Check any travel arrangements again. Don't give up! You've done the work!
- On the day before, focus on getting rest and go through your 'the day before the exam' file. Do not look at any new material.
- Spend time thinking about how you are going to tackle the day – get a strategy and remind yourself of all the hard work that has got you to this point.
- Give it your absolute best on the day. Be prepared. Avoid frameshift errors.
- Look at each question carefully, and stick to time. Move on from really tricky questions that are holding you up.
- Good luck. May the force be with you.

10

After the Exam

We all walked out of the exam in a daze, dazzled by the sunlight, disbelieving that a year of work was all over. Waiting for the exam results to come out was the weirdest week. I was absolutely convinced that I'd failed, had reorganised my desk, bought four more packets of felt pens, started a brand new colour-coded study timetable and decided which study course to go on.

If you can take it from people not exactly known for their relaxed demeanours, *try* and chill out after the exam; remember that the College can't fail everyone.

What to Do If You Pass

Congratulations! People will stop you in the corridors of the hospital and shake your hand. You will achieve demigod-like status to the registrars the year below you. Your consultants will be pleased as punch. Please turn to Chapter 13, which will encourage you to celebrate and have a short break before starting to prepare for the Clinical Exam.

What to Do If You Don't Pass

Failing is just awful. If you are at our centre, please come by the office and we will make you a cup of tea, proffer tissues and nod gently. For everyone else, find a sympathetic ear, and turn immediately to Chapter 30 for advice written by a battle-weary soul who has walked in your shoes and gone on to success.

How to Pass the RACP Written and Clinical Exams: The Insider's Guide,
Second Edition. Zoë Raos and Cheryl Johnson.
© 2017 John Wiley & Sons Ltd. Published 2017 by John Wiley & Sons Ltd.

Section 2

The Clinical Exam

11

Introduction to the FRACP Clinical Exam

Passing the FRACP Written Exam gave us a wonderful feeling of bewildering, euphoric disbelief. We spent a few days in the pub comforting our unsuccessful colleagues and congratulating our successful ones. This glorious feeling lasted for a few days and then it slowly began to dawn on us – we were only halfway through. There was still the Clinical Exam to go!

Our happy cloud quickly dissolved into fear and despair. We realised we didn't even know what a long case was. To make matters worse, there were no comforting words from our seniors – they gleefully let us in on the worst/best kept secret in medicine:

The Clinical is worse than the Written.

Then, the truth became apparent.

- Knowledge evaporates in an exponential fashion as soon as the Written Exam is over. By the end of the first week, we could barely remember our own names let alone the difference between pANCA and cANCA.
- We were complete mental, physical and emotional wrecks after the Written Exam. To start working towards another exam was an horrendous proposition.
- We'd trained our brains to work in multi-choice format, which is the exact opposite way to approach the Clinical Exam.
- Unlike the Written, where swotting is done in privacy and mistakes are our own, preparing for the Clinical involves ritual humiliation in front of respected colleagues. We got used to seeing faces filled with shock and disbelief at how useless we were. At one point, we

How to Pass the RACP Written and Clinical Exams: The Insider's Guide,
Second Edition. Zoë Raos and Cheryl Johnson.
© 2017 John Wiley & Sons Ltd. Published 2017 by John Wiley & Sons Ltd.

wondered if anonymous phone calls might be made to the Medical Council about our competence to practise.

Don't freak out yet! Despite all this doom and gloom, we also discovered:

- somehow, you become desensitised to the humiliation and take criticism on the chin. We are now perfectly trained to compete on a range of reality TV shows
- a mixture of humility, confidence, knowledge and experience is what separates the girls/boys from the women/men, both on the day and in real life (in other words, it was probably good for us).

We don't want to imply in any way that the Written Exam was a push-over. Memorising renal histology is a soul-destroying and tedious process. That said, on the day of the Written Exam, you could rock up in comfy tracky daks, 2B pencil in hand, and get to work making the best guesses you can. If you make a mistake, it is a personal experience between a candidate and an exam paper. It's a stressful day, to be sure, but not humiliating. The Clinical Exam is a whole different beast. The examiner is real, standing in front of you, asking curly questions and looking bemused at your answers. Suddenly, passing seems to hinge on hiding that quivering mess of insecurity and pretending to be a confident and all-knowing doctor.

The Clinical Exam is a game. You need to train, get yourself in shape, have the right attitude and know as much about the opposition as you can. Athletes train for years for the Olympics – they look forward to their competing event with nervous excitement and determination to win. Think of yourself as an Olympic athlete but with only a couple of months to train.

Upcoming changes

The possibility of a twice-yearly Written Exam may extend to the possibility of twice-yearly Clinical Exams too. Since the dawn of time, the Clinical Exam has been held three months after the Written with a little bit more time for the Aussies. Candidates do two long cases and four short cases. It is carved thus on a stone tablet in Sydney. Change will come one day so keep in close contact with the RACP to see if any potential changes could affect you directly in the year you plan to sit.

Why Is There a Clinical Exam?

The College knows now that you know your facts. What it is assessing you for are clinical skills, attitudes and interpersonal relationships. The exam itself is fairly valid and reliable as an assessment tool. That said, every year, just like in the Written, good candidates who do the work and deserve to pass have a bad day, fail and have to wait another year. We want to help you have a good day, or at least an OK day, and pass this exam.

Getting Your Timing Right: When to Sit the Clinical Exam

The College will send you a pile of information (also on the website) about eligibility to sit the Clinical Exam. Most registrars who successfully pass the Written Exam in March are eligible to sit the Clinical Exam in June (New Zealand) or July (Australia) of the same year. This gives you 12–16 weeks to prepare.

In the bad old days, a successful Written Exam candidate had two attempts at the Clinical. If he or she failed both these attempts, the candidate would have to study for the Written Exam all over again. From 2017, new trainees are allowed three attempts at the Written, and three attempts at the Clinical. Check the College website for the transition plan for candidates who started training pre-2017. We implore you, for your own sake, do not take these attempts lightly! Turn to chapter 30 for a deeper understanding of Snakes and Ladders if you need more convincing. Do your best to pass the Clinical Exam the first time round.

Summary

- The Clinical Exam is worse than the Written.
- One good thing is that the pain is relatively short-lived – it will all be over in 12–16 weeks.
- If you are eligible, fill in the paperwork and send the RACP your credit card details to confirm your place on exam day.
- These 3–4 months will be incredibly intense, and involve asking for help from respected seniors and then making a complete idiot of yourself.
- Despite all of this, it is very possible to pass with the right preparation, attitude, help and advice.

12

The Clinical Exam Marking Schedule

The Clinical Exam consists of two long cases and four short cases. The day is divided into two sessions, each session containing one long and two short cases, with a lunch break in the middle.

Exam Day

Morning session
Two short cases
One long case

Lunch break (where no one really eats that much)

Afternoon session
One long case
Two short cases

The Mathematics of Passing the Clinical Exam

Just like knowing how to do a Punnet square and knowing you've got 1.6 minutes per question for the Written, know your Clinical Exam arithmetic.

A short case is worth seven marks = 28 marks total for the four short cases.

A long case is also marked out of seven, but the mark is multiplied by 3 = 42 marks for two long cases. Forty percent of your grade will be

How to Pass the RACP Written and Clinical Exams: The Insider's Guide,
Second Edition. Zoë Raos and Cheryl Johnson.
© 2017 John Wiley & Sons Ltd. Published 2017 by John Wiley & Sons Ltd.

based on short cases and 60% on long cases. Practising for short cases helps your long cases a lot. You must pass at least one long case and one short case to pass the exam.

Half-Marks: 'Plus and Minus'

In recent years, to allow the examiner to give the candidate the benefit of the doubt, half-marks have been instituted. For example, a highly nervous candidate might fluff up and forget to check for a water-hammer pulse but makes the correct diagnosis of aortic regurgitation in a short case. The discussion is faltering, with the examiners dragging out every point, but the candidate is nice to the patient, gets the answers correct and interprets the chest X-ray correctly. This candidate would get 4+, or a 5– (same score of 4.5). Or, let's say that a long case patient has to leave for a 15-minute toilet break right in the middle of the history. The candidate does not give up, gets the opening gambit and the start of the problem list lined up during the loo break. Once the patient is back, the candidate keeps going, takes an abbreviated social history and does a targeted examination. When the examiners ask 'Were there any difficulties?', the candidate explains about the toilet break, then moves on and presents the long case as best they can, touching on areas in the history and examination cut short by the loo break. Then, he/she keeps going with an excellent summary and problem list followed by a focused discussion (worked on during that 15 minutes with the information available). The examiners agree that the candidate did an excellent job, but the 15 minutes did mean that key parts of the social and past medical history were missing. The candidate gets 5+ rather than 5.

A word of warning – the 'Were there any difficulties?' question is a fraught one. This is not an opportunity to have a whinge about how poor an historian the patient was.

Red Dots and Supplementary Cases

If the patient spent 35 minutes in the loo or got chest pain or ran out of the room crying after a text message, or anything occurred that majorly affected a candidate's ability to complete the case, on Exam Day the examiners put a 'red dot' on the candidate's marking sheet. Any 'red dots' are taken into account in the candidate's overall mark.

Depending on the candidate's performance on the day, along with the seriousness of the 'interruption/difficulties' faced by the candidate in the case, the candidate may be asked to do a supplementary case on a later day.

Adding Up the Marks

Your total score is then multiplied by 3, making the highest total possible score 210. Like the Glasgow Coma Scale, there are no 'zero' marks.

You need 120/210 marks to pass. The College came up with this multiplication method to spread out the bell curve of candidates. What follows are detailed marking schedules adapted from the official RACP sheets that examiners use.

Permutations of the Marking Scheme

Hopefully the following maths exercise will demonstrate that you must spend time on short case and long case preparation, and that keeping cool under pressure can make the difference between passing and failing.

Scenario	Short 1	Short 2	Short 3	Short 4	Long 1	Long 2	Result
Jo Average	4+	4	4	4	4(12)	4+ (13.5)	153 – pass
Long case one-trick pony	2	3	2	3	5(15)	5(15)	120 – fail
Skating on thin ice	2	3	2	5	4(12)	4(12)	108 – fail
Lucky long case	3	3	3	4	5(15)	4(12)	120 – pass
Unlucky long case with exam nerves	6	5	5	5	2(6)	4(12)	117 – fail
Unlucky long case but kept calm under pressure	6	4+	5	5	3(9)	4 + (13.5)	129 – pass

Long case Marking Schedule

	History	Examination	Synthesis	Insight	Management
1	No structure to history. Superficial with details	No structure to examination	Most issues not identified or prioritised	No attempt to recognise impact of disease	Unable to interpret investigations. Unable to formulate management plan
2	Poorly presented history. Missed out key points. Disorganised	Missed significant physical signs	Needed a lot of prompting to establish a problem list	Didn't recognise most aspects of the disease and impact on patient and family. Didn't take life-lines	Difficulty interpreting investigations and poor management plan
3	Left out key parts of history	Missed some important physical signs but found others	Poor prioritisation of problems. Had a problem list, but not in the right order	Didn't recognise all aspects of disease and its impact on patient and family	Errors interpreting investigations. Disorganised approach to requesting investigations. Management plan lacks confidence
4	Complete history	Found all the signs	Thorough problem list	Understands impact of disease (physical and psychological) as well as effect the treatment and prognosis has on patient and family	Appropriate interpretation of investigation results. Sensible and balanced. Recognises adverse effects of treatment
5	Complete history with emphasis on most important aspects	Found all the signs plus relative negatives	Thorough problem list divided into more important and less important issues	Empathetically explores subtle issues impacting on patient and family	Thorough and appropriate management plan with insight into impact of the disease
6	Complete history with empathetic extraction of the 'hidden gold'	Finds all the signs plus subtle signs that support diagnosis	Finds all major and minor problems, carefully prioritised	Maturely conveys subtle and difficult aspects of functioning. Demonstrates balance and sophistication with social support	Thorough management plan with discussion of long-term impact
7	Exceptional history	Perfect examination	Excellent problem list with understanding of how problems interact	Complete, thorough understanding of psychological and social aspects	Excellent management plan with discussion of prognosis

Short case Marking Schedule

	Approach	Technique	Accuracy	Interpretation of signs	Investigations
1	Inappropriate, rude and insensitive	Unable to complete an appropriate examination	Missed everything	No diagnosis made. Unable to respond to any prompting	Unable to suggest reasonable investigations and misinterprets what is given
2	Hurt the patient, examiners had to step in	Didn't finish in time. Needed substantial examiner intervention	Missed major signs and found signs that were not there (fibbed and fudged)	Unable to suggest diagnosis, goes down the wrong track, life-lines not taken	Unable to use investigations to assist in diagnosis. Inappropriate dependence on investigations
3	Hurt the patient	Needs prompting to proceed with examination	Missed some major signs, didn't include important negatives	Difficulty interpreting signs. More than minor prompting, recognised life-lines. Differential diagnosis scanty or poor	Needs prompting to receive investigations. Some correct interpretation. When given investigations, complains about quality
4	Introduces self. Respectful of modesty and of discomfort	Good, confident examination, in time frame, fluent. Can think on feet and adapt the exam according to signs found	Found major signs, including significant negatives	Appropriate interpretation of signs. Formulates a reasonable and sensible diagnosis. Gives a good differential diagnosis. A little prompting OK	Asks for the correct investigations results, can interpret correctly and relate back to the patient's findings. Minor prompting OK in a complex case
5	As above	As above	Found major and minor signs, including relevant negatives	Identifies most likely diagnosis, justifies it and a sensible differential diagnosis list	Correctly interprets all major findings as above
6	As above	As above	As above	As above, with an excellent differential	As above, and can integrate findings with insightfulness and no prompting
7	As above	As above	Found absolutely what the examiners did, perhaps more	Nails it. Discusses alternative diagnoses at a consultant level	Thorough, integrated approach and understands subtleties. Recognises areas of doubt at a consultant level

- **Jo Average**: clear pass. No outstanding performances but no disasters either. Joe Average kept her head, had a couple of good moments where the examiners' benefit of the doubt was deployed, and those little 'plus' half-marks popped her from a nail-biting 120 to a comfortable 153.
- **Long case one-trick pony**: this candidate put his eggs in one basket and practised heaps of long cases, and left short cases to chance on the day. You must pass one short case to pass. See you next year.
- **Skating on thin ice**: this candidate failed three-quarters of her shorts. Solid passes in the longs were not enough to save her.
- **Lucky long case**: one 5/7 in a single long case allowed this candidate some breathing room on the shorts – he passed comfortably.
- **Unlucky long case with exam nerves**: even nailing all the short cases could not save this candidate from the effects of a badly failed long case. Her nerves meant she didn't recognise life-lines. Hard luck.
- **Unlucky long case but kept calm under pressure**: unlike the previous candidate, this guy somehow managed to drag that terrible morning long case up to a 3/7; the afternoon case went much better with an extra 'plus' half-mark. Clear pass.

In all the scenarios, successful candidates almost always passed both their long cases. The adage 'You can never fail a long but you can muff up some shorts' is reasonably accurate. You may be able to get by with a borderline fail in a long case if you nail everything else, but you won't survive a badly failed long case.

Hopefully, this exercise will show you that the Clinical Exam is really easy to pass. It is also really easy to fail. Every mark counts but the long case marks are three times as important. The only difference between the last two candidates was the ability to cope with pressure. Instead of crumbling and giving up, the last candidate didn't lose his cool, remembered to perform a diabetic foot examination and made a good case for not starting warfarin even with a high CHA2DS2-VASc score. He also admitted that he didn't know an answer instead of lying about it, which is a good way of deploying the examiner's benefit of the doubt.

Paeds Point
This marking schedule is identical for you. Using the example of the last two candidates, 'Exam Nerves' was terrified by an adolescent who wouldn't talk to her. 'Kept Calm' did the best HEEADSSS assessment he could muster with this recalcitrant teenager with lupus whose mum left in a huff halfway through. The teen didn't take out her earphones and minimally co-operated with the examination. 'Kept Calm' expressed that it was a difficult case in the discussion without whinging and gave a sensible strategy for extracting more information from the GP, school and previous specialist. He also had some excellent, practical suggestions for improving the young person's relationship with healthcare services, and pointed out how challenging the transition of her care would prove to be. Know this: You will *automatically fail* a short or long case if you hurt a child or young person. You will also fail if you cannot come up with a watertight child protection plan if concerns are raised about safety. A vague 'I would refer to child protection' is not enough to pass – the candidate must have a good working understanding of the systems and legalities. It is perfectly fine if you are examined in a different geographical area to use your local procedures in the discussion.

How Do The Examiners Know What a Pass Is?

As inserting microchips into the brains of the examiners would never get ethics approval, the examiners are all calibrated the day before the exam with candidate videos. There are two candidate videos shown – one long case and one short case. These videos are shown across Australasia to ensure there is consistency. All examiners and organisers watch each video and then mark the candidate. This is followed by a small group discussion about the case and what the mark should be.

On the day, once the candidate leaves the room, both examiners mark the candidate individually using the standardised marking schedule. Following that, both examiners discuss the marks they gave and come to a consensus. Believe it or not, calibration works 99%

of the time as marks are often identical, give or take half a mark. Occasionally, there is a significant disagreement, in which case rank is pulled and the most experienced examiner present has the final say.

Summary

- Money for jam marks in the Clinical: don't hurt the patient. Introduce yourself. Thank them at the end.
- Know the standard you are aiming for by reading the marking schedule. Know what a 4/7 mark means in both a short case and a long case.
- + marks are given when the examiner's benefit of the doubt is deployed. These half-marks make a big difference.
- Keeping your cool makes all the difference between passing and failing on the day.
- When practising, make a copy of the marking schedule (in the appendix) so practice examiners can mark you accurately.
- Examiners are calibrated carefully. On Exam Day the actual marking is fair and accurate.

13

Two Weeks of Ground Work

Now you know a bit about the Clinical, it's time to burn your Written Exam track pants, stop thinking in multi-guess format and start acting like a junior consultant. It takes time to recover from the Written to avoid burnout – we reckon two weeks is about right. Be smart, and use this recovery time to tick off some important tasks.

- Organise a **celebration dinner** with study buddies, friends, family and anyone else who supported you for the Written Exam. It's time to re-enlist the troops for the next round and thank them for their support thus far.
- Book yourself into a **Clinical Exam preparation course** and any **mock exams.**
- Sort out the contents of your **new kit bag.**
- **Appearance is vital**. Go through your wardrobe. Think about what you could wear on the day (see page 98). Go shopping.
- **Buy the books** that you need (see page 92).
- **Organise study leave**, as much as you sensibly can. Make sure that you are not on night duty the week before the Exam. Swap your shifts if you need to.
- **Buy a diary** to book cases or use a calendar function on your smartphone. Aim to book two long cases and at least three short case sessions per week.
- **Start contacting practice examiners** (see page 106 for the different types of practice examiners). Emailing worked well for us. Email current and past examiners, consultants and post exam registrars from your hospital or any other hospital you've worked at, explain you've just passed the Written and that you would very

How to Pass the RACP Written and Clinical Exams: The Insider's Guide,
Second Edition. Zoë Raos and Cheryl Johnson.
© 2017 John Wiley & Sons Ltd. Published 2017 by John Wiley & Sons Ltd.

much appreciate some help with Clinical prep. Talk to your DPT about organised sessions at your hospital. Consultants have limited pockets of time to take candidates for cases, so best to book ahead.

- **Make a 'To do'** list of short and long cases you want to do. This will help to identify any obvious holes in your knowledge and experience to date. You may, for example, need to spend a day at the regional transplant centre or rheumatology clinic, so start planning this now.
- **Start socialising and exercising again.** People skills and healthy energy are needed to pass the Clinical. Expand your horizons, cast off that exam pallor. Go to the movies. Take in a concert! Reintegrate into the real world.
- **Book into preparation courses** – see page 96. There are some excellent courses for adult medicine candidates – they are popular and oversubscribed so register now.

Three Key Parts to Passing the Clinical Exam

A late great professor spent many years passing and failing candidates. He described three key parts to passing the Clinical Exam.

1) Your innate ability as a doctor.
2) Luck on the day.
3) The amount and quality of practice you put in.

You have to have all three parts to pass the exam well. Two out of three makes it hard to pass, one out of the three means failing is guaranteed.

Your Innate Ability as a Doctor

Being a good doctor helps but is not enough to pass this exam. If you count yourself among this esteemed group, do not make the mistake of many before you and rely only on your personal abilities. Many outstanding, brilliant, thoroughly superb clinicians have failed this exam due to bad luck and inadequate preparation.

Others fail because they are superb junior registrars but are just not up to the senior trainee standard which is expected on Exam Day, usually because they sit the Clinical Exam too soon.

Luck on the Day

Many say that you make your own luck, which is true. Nonetheless, every year excellent candidates crash and burn when faced with obscure pathologies, recalcitrant patients, tough examiners, mind blanks and tears. This could happen to anyone. While luck can very much go against you, it can also go your way. We will discuss disaster patients, how to steel your nerves and how to turn adversity into triumph (or, at least, a half-mark).

The Amount of Practice You Put In

This third factor is something that you can do something about. A senior doctor (who makes us nervous because he is so super-smart) admitted that when he was a registrar, he thought that all you had to do to pass the exam was be a good doctor and turn up. He failed. The second year, he practised playing the game and saying all the right things. This time he passed. Hopefully, this book will give you some idea how to approach this practice and mean that you will look slick and polished on the day.

How to Get Humble and Ask for Help

The FRACP Clinical Exam is bored indelibly into the minds of anyone who has ever attempted it. No-one ever forgets how difficult it was to prepare, how essential it was to practise in front of seniors, or how stressful the actual day was. If you give people enough notice and ask nicely, most seniors are incredibly generous with their time and advice.

Asking for practice sessions is a cap-in-hand experience. Asking for help pales in comparison to being a complete bumbling, fumbling drongo during the practice session itself. It takes immense amounts of grit and masochistic tendencies to ask to be humiliated. Remarkably, horrendous displays of ignorance, disorganisation and stuttering are generally forgotten by consultants and not held against you forever more (especially if you go on to pass).

You cannot pass the Clinical Exam on your own. The amount of actual organisation candidates do is incredibly variable from work-place to workplace. Some hospitals have chief residents who arrange all the short and long case sessions for all the candidates. Other hospitals have no such luck, so candidates are on their own.

- Get together with all the other Clinical Exam candidates in your hospital. If you're the only one, get in touch with candidates in your region. You cannot do this alone. Get an email list, form a rag-tag study group, meet regularly and share details of good cases in a way that is up to date and respects patient privacy in accordance with the rules of your institution.
- Organise your own weekly short case sessions with your local and regional candidates, ideally with a supervising senior registrar or consultant.
- Amass an army of friendly consultants and advanced trainees to whom you can present cases. You may have worked with them before, or not. It doesn't matter. Ask.
- When we say 'share cases', we mean it. The disturbing, tedious and unphysicianly behaviour of candidates deliberately not sharing cases with others does not give anyone an advantage on Exam Day.
- Ask your friendly local -ologist when their clinics are run, and go along.
- Even in smaller centres, there will be examiners in your region. Word of mouth and local knowledge will tell you who they are. Book in long and short case sessions with examiners.
- Know the limitations and gaps in your knowledge and training. Seek out sessions in other hospitals (for example, neurology, HIV, transplant, rheumatology). You will have to cold-call or cold-email consultants or advanced trainees in these specialised places. Explain your situation; most of the time there will be someone who can help you attend an outpatient clinic, find some cases or (BAZINGA!) feel sorry for you and take you for a couple of cases.

The Kit Bag

Start assembling your kit bag early, and take it proudly with you to all your short and long case sessions. You will get used to it and learn where all the gear lives. Most gear is easy to find or borrow, except for red hat-pins. There must be some sadist who buys up all the red hat-pins in haberdasheries across Australasia every March. You can order hat-pins online from www.hatpinsdirect.co.uk or www.usneurologicals.com; otherwise, a tongue depressor with a red sticky dot on the end works just fine. Despite one of the authors toying with a little pink number with fur trim, kit bags end up black and conservative.

In recent years, we have observed the move from minimalistic slim-line travel wallets to the 'little black briefcase' (ironically named since some of these briefcases are bigger than the candidates). While the choice of accessories is up to you, a kit bag just needs to be big enough to fit your gear and be at your fingertips. You don't want to waste valuable short case time unzipping your bag or fumbling around looking for cotton wool. Examiners have looked on with bemusement at the increasing sophistication and complexity of the 'little black briefcase' and beware of the examiner who adjusts the combination lock during a mock exam when you're not looking.

Pictured below are the options for your kit bag. Also, put your stethoscope in your bag or pocket. While we sling stethoscopes around our necks daily, it is better to have it in your kit bag for practice and on the day.

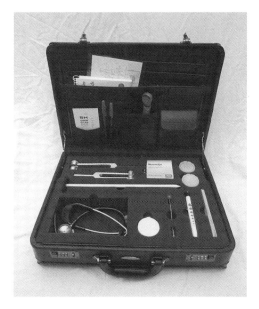

Briefcase

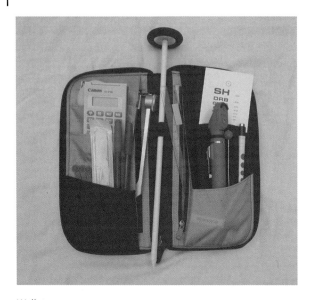

Wallet

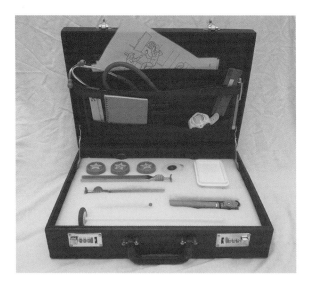

Paediatric bag

> **Paeds Point**
>
> For the developmental assessment, your stuff must be easily accessible to you but completely inaccessible to your small, curious patient. We recommend a soft bag. Divide up your items so you are able to pull things out like a magician. A briefcase (as pictured) can work, but beware that kids may immediately open it and pull out all the good stuff. Start with a toy that is interesting … but not too interesting. If you put in your prized Matchbox car collection, you will never see it again. Prising your vintage Batmobile out of a howling small child's fingers as the bell goes is not what you want to do after a long case. Something cheap, safe, small and squeaky or with a light will do just fine. Give stickers as a reward at the end. They should be pre-cut and offer a limited choice ('Star sticker or firetruck sticker?') or you will never leave the room!

Suggested gear for your kit bag

	Adults	Paeds
Tendon hammer (nice and springy and not those detestable metal retracting ones)	✔	✔
Neuro-tips/safety pins (unlikely to need in the Paeds exam but present with a flourish then put away)	✔	✔
Cotton wool	✔	✔
Wooden spatula (can be broken in half for pinprick sensation)	✔	✔
Pocket torch with new batteries	✔	✔
Ophthalmoscope that you know how to use	✔	
Tuning forks 128 Hz for vibration sensation testing 256 Hz for Weber's test (optional) 512 Hz for Rinne's test (can be used for Weber's too)	✔	✔
Ruler or tape measure (height/weight charts for Paeds should be provided)	✔	✔
Stethoscope	✔	✔
Paper and pen for testing handwriting and sentences/drawing	✔	
Jar with coin and key for hand function and astereognosis	✔	
Hand-held visual acuity chart/picture visual acuity charts	✔	✔
Red hat-pin or tongue depressor with a red sticky dot at the end	✔	✔

	Adults	Paeds
Stopwatch for timing short and long cases	✔	✔
Boston Cookie Theft picture for aphasia testing	✔	
Detailed picture books for language development		✔
Coloured pens/crayons and paper for patient drawing		✔
Small ball for gross motor skills		✔
Picture cards for testing language and naming		✔
Picture cards for testing receptive language – sitting, eating, drinking, running, sleeping		✔
Coloured blocks for fine motor skills		✔
Soft toy that is not too interesting (no cars)		✔
Red ring with a string		✔
Simple jigsaw puzzles with shapes		✔
Raisins or cake sprinkles for visual assessment, co-ordination and pincer grip		✔
Small bottle of hand sanitiser	✔	✔

Adult medicine physicians are openly jealous that our paediatric colleagues get to use cake sprinkles and crayons in their kit bags.

Leave your mobile phone in the hotel or at home. Mobile devices of any kind are not permitted during the exam.

Book Reviews

Unlike the Written Exam, where your desk groaned under a comforting pile of journals and textbooks, the Clinical Exam doesn't need a vast array of reference materials. No amount of reading will take the place of getting out there and practising on patients.

Essential Texts

Adult Medicine trainees must buy both the Talley and O'Connors, read them cover to cover, make notes and read them carefully after each case. The other books are less compulsory but can be useful. It is a good idea to canvas previous registrars to borrow their books before deciding to purchase them.

For paediatric trainees, *Examination Paediatrics* is your go-to essential text.

Read on for reviews of essential texts, and other books that candidates have found useful. They are a positive use of your time on those rainy Sunday afternoons when you know there is work to do but you just can't face another patient.

Clinical Examination: A Systematic Guide to Physical Diagnosis, 7th edition (Talley and O'Connor)

This is the Bible when it comes to examination technique. What was medicine like before these guys came along? This book is densely written and meticulously detailed, with humour sprinkled through to lighten the load. The T&O exam technique is the gold standard – this is what examiners expect on the day. It's a good starting point to make sure you examine in the same order that this book suggests. We recommend reading T&O early on and re-reading it several times before the Big Day.

Examination Medicine: A Guide to Physician Training, 6th edition (Talley and O'Connor)

This second, slightly smaller book is written specifically for the Clinical Exam. It describes plenty of typical long cases with key learning points. It also goes through common short cases in each specialty. Overall, it's a goldmine of detail and excellent for lugging around for short case practice, so whoever is acting as examiner can grill with authority. Any textbook can get out of date, but while - pesky-mabs come and go, how to do a solid cardiovascular exam will never go out of style.

An Aid to the MRCP PACES: Volume 1: Stations 1 and 3, 4th edition (Ryder et al.)

This used to be one book but is now divided into three separate volumes. You want Volume 1, as Stations 1 and 3 are those that most resemble the FRACP short cases. The other volumes cover material on the MRCP that isn't directly examined in our Clinical Exam. Its main use is short case preparation.

This gem of a book takes you through suggested examination techniques, and then has practice cases for you to review. The MRCP books are great for the presentation part of a short case.

Best of all are the 'records' which are scripts of what to say if you come across a patient with, say, interstitial lung disease.

250 Cases in Clinical Medicine, 4th edition (Baliga)

250 Cases is another British book useful for your short cases. It is less prescriptive in terms of actual presentation style than Ryder but has more fine detail about each case. It contains some questions and answers, some of which are relevant to the FRACP exam (signs of severity of mitral stenosis, indications for surgery, etc.). As with any book from overseas, check that medical management is the same as the local guidelines. Good as a reference for reading up about the specific details of a particular case after long or short case practice.

Neurological Clinical Examination: A Concise Guide (Morris and Jankovic)

This is an updated version of *The Neurological Short Case* written by Australian neurologists. It's easy to read with lots of pictures. It also presents chapters of cases that you are likely to encounter in the exam ('This man has foot drop, please examine') with logical explanations of how to examine a patient and work out the diagnosis. It is the only book that made neurology make sense for us. Also comes with more than 100 video clips accessed by QR code demonstrating everything from Parinaud's syndrome to spastic quadriparesis. Gold.

Aids to the Examination of the Peripheral Nervous System, 5th edition (O'Brien)

This nice, short book has lots of photographs to help you work out how to examine individual muscles and nerve groups. It describes excellent examination techniques for the upper and lower limbs, and contains nice pictures of myotomes and dermatomes.

Mastering the Medical Long Case, 2nd edition (Jayasinghe)

This well-written book is not too long, and is written specifically about the FRACP exam. Many candidates find this book illuminating, particularly seeing practice cases structured into a logical format. It also makes an excellent effort at going through common long cases (e.g. diabetes, transplant, heart failure), with descriptions of the major issues, investigations and likely questions that crop up. It's definitely worth getting your hands on, even if you just borrow it for a weekend and flick through it.

> ### Paeds Point
>
> ***Examination Paediatrics*, 4th edition (Harris)** This is the book that paediatric registrars in our part of the world use as a text to prepare for the Clinical, and was originally inspired by T&O. Any book that quotes the obscure SciFi series *Red Dwarf* has got to be good (in a previous edition). Common long and short cases are described for each major area of paediatrics. Like T&O, this book is very heavy on detail, so can be quite exhausting reading after a long day's work, but has a healthy sprinkling of humour to get the reader through. It is useful to lug around during practice short cases for the grilling session. The actual method of presentation may not perfectly suit all candidates, but it is an excellent place to start.
>
> ***The FRACP Paediatric Clinical Exam*** – self-published by the Royal Children's Hospital & Monash Medical Centre, Melbourne
> This is 25 A4 pages of pure gold. This free online book has been handed down from chief resident to chief resident with upgrades on the way. It is filled with mnemonics, survival tips for both short and long cases and (beyond gold) there are three A4 pages written by examiners describing why candidates pass … and why they fail. There are some excellent psychological tips for surviving the preparation and the Big Day itself. Worth a quick read-through for adult medicine trainees too. Fantastic. Best found using Google, or using this link: http://www.rch.org.au/uploadedFiles/Main/Content/medicaleducation/Clinical%20Exam%20Handbook%20RCH%202013.pdf

Course Reviews

In recent years, specialised courses have come on the market to help candidates prepare for the exam. They are by no means compulsory but you may want to consider them.

Tauranga Neurology Course

The two-day Neurology Course in Tauranga has been running for many years and is always well attended. Neurologists are aware that their specialty bamboozles outsiders; this course seems to be their way of educating the unwashed masses. A gentle reminder – do not rely solely on this course for your neurology preparation. It was much more useful to be well practised in the upper/lower limb and cranial nerve examinations, know which end of the ophthalmoscope to use and to have read through the relevant chapters in T&O before attending the course.

The first day consists of introductory lectures outlining an approach to the different neurology exams. The second day is where the real action is, dividing into small groups round-robin style, with candidates taking turns to examine real neurology cases and present their findings to neurologists from around the country. Most of the tutors keep their advice to a FRACP rather than Professor of Neurology level.

Unless you work in a neurology department, you will never see as many weird and wonderful cases, let alone this close to the exam. This may be the only chance you get to see a case of lateral medullary syndrome or intranuclear ophthalmoplegia other than on Exam Day.

Everyone we've spoken to who attended this course came away with a better understanding of neurology. You may feel completely humiliated in the presence of some of the best neurologists in the country but better now than meeting them during the exam.

Website: www.neurologybop.co.nz/course.htm

DeltaMed Clinical Exam Course

This is a well-organised, efficient, one-day course run by the same crowd who put on the DeltaMed two-week Melbourne Written Exam course. While they do go through short case techniques, the main focus is on long case mark maximisation. It is based on fast analysis of information given by the patient and how to use it in formulating a case summary, problem list and investigations, treatments and solutions. Candidates who have done this course found these skills to be valuable, especially for study group work. They re-presented, critiqued and discussed the long cases of the week with each other.

There are no real live patients to practise on, so if you are still struggling to extract information, your time may be better spent in the hospitals. It was particularly good for those of us who could get all the information from the patients but had problems synthesising and summarising the information into a coherent format. Time was split between effective, informative lectures and small group sessions with tutors, where the attendees would practise turning a standard blathering rant of information into clear, structured presentations with a prioritised problem list. They also ran through key topics to have under your belt (e.g. diabetes).

Some attendees thought it made the difference between passing and failing. Almost everyone who attended thought it was excellent. There is online self-directed study material to complete prior to the course.

Website: www.deltamed.com.au

Dunedin Clinical Course

This intensive, successful and oversubscribed seven-day clinical exam preparation course has been held in Dunedin for nearly a decade. This course is efficient and well organised. Priority is given to local Dunedin candidates and folk who have failed the Clinical before.

Previous attenders describe introductory lectures that outline a general approach to the exam, including demonstrations of good (and bad) long case and short case presentations. The remaining days focused on the individual specialty exams. Candidates were divided into small groups, and cases were done under exam conditions while 'examiners' acted their part by marking you silently as you examined. The real strength was the sheer number and variety of cases presented.

All the organisers in Dunedin understood the marking schedule and the standards expected for the exam. Each case was marked and discussed, meaning candidates gained a real feel for what a passing (and failing) performance felt like. Experts quickly corrected bad examination techniques for both short and long cases. The feedback was constructive. If you are a repeat sitter, we thoroughly encourage you to apply.

Website: www.otago.ac.nz/dsm-medicine/postgraduate/professional-education

> **Paeds Point: Organised courses – the lack thereof**
>
> If you are an enterprising paeds person, there is a big gap in the market. As far as we are aware, there are no extracurricular courses for paediatric trainees preparing for the Clinical Exam. The exam is difficult enough to organise in paediatrics (co-ordinating parents, siblings, childcare, school, small pool of well-known patients …) so mock exams don't exist. Paeds trainees are reliant on the quality of the teaching programmes at individual hospitals. Thankfully, paediatric trainees and consultants are usually co-operative and helpful, and often trainees from smaller centres can join in with sessions at the tertiary/quaternary centres.

Personal Appearance – First Impressions Count

There are plenty of candidates who have worn their own style on Exam Day and, because they are great doctors, the examiners overlooked their questionable sartorial choices but had a good giggle at the paisley flares and platform shoes at the examiners' dinner. One candidate had his wife clip his dreadlocks to a uniform 30 cm, tied them back neatly with a hair-tie, and he passed. Other candidates feel their best in a conservative outfit from their country of origin, perhaps a smart shalwar kameez for Indian women or a puletasi for a Samoan man. The key is to look smart, to be clean and groomed, to be able to undertake the task at hand and to be comfortable. It is very important that your appearance reflects who you are and does not detract from your performance on the day. Remember, in everyday working life, we need to gain the trust of our patients and our team, and personal appearance and first impressions are crucial.

A smart outfit and impeccable personal hygiene make you feel more legitimate as an exam candidate in your practice sessions and on the day. Importantly, a smart outfit will not distract the examiners from your clinical skills. Overwhelming body odour, greasy hair, dandruff, an ill-fitting suit, a short tight skirt or a stained novelty tie mean a candidate has to overcome a lot of preconceptions. If someone can see up it, down it or through it, forget it. Make it simple – look smart.

Start wearing your clothes, haircut, shoes and make-up well before the exam, as you'll look and be more comfortable on the day. A panic-stricken shopping mission and bad haircut the night before the

Clinical never ends well, so plan your outfit well ahead. Make sure you can walk, everything stays put, the clothes fit well, you look good, you feel comfortable and you have full use of both shoulder girdles for doing a neurological exam.

Advice for Men

- **Clean shoes with matching socks** – you can't go wrong with nice shiny lace-up black leather shoes that have been worn in but are clean and polished. Cheap shoes stand out a mile.
- **Smart shirt** with a non-strangling collar in a conservative colour like white, pale blue or a subtle check. Leave anything that could induce a migraine at home. Have a couple of spare shirts handy in case your three-year-old daughter covers you with ketchup on Exam Day morning. In the UK, you can fail a Clinical Exam by not having your shirt rolled up to elbow height! This has not quite reached Australasia but is probably coming. Take a spare shirt to change into halfway through the day in case of sudden hyperhydrosis.
- **Trousers** – make sure these fit well, perfectly match your jacket if you're wearing one and are hemmed for your height. Trousers that are too tight make it difficult to sit (for the long case) and manoeuvre (for the shorts). Trousers that are too big look silly. Lots of men in recent years forewent suits and stuck with a shirt-tie-trouser combination (and passed).
- **Suit jacket** – make sure this is well-fitted. Examiners can spot a suit that is too big or small from a hundred paces. Darker suits are better, as they are regarded as being more conservative, show fewer marks and are more forgiving for sweat stains.
- **Tie** – if you want to wear a tie, it must be conservative, match your suit and be controlled with a tie-pin (flapping your tie in the patient's face is not a good look in the short case). In this day and age of infection control, the tie has been maligned as a carrier of pestilence and plague. Examiners in Australasia still seem to like ties on blokes. If you don't wear a tie, make sure the rest of your outfit is smart and presentable. Bow ties are becoming increasingly popular, but perhaps not on Exam Day.
- Get a **haircut** the week before. Make sure hair is clean and washed. If you have long hair, tie it neatly back. If you have a beard, get it trimmed and tidied.
- **Avoid** earrings and gimmicky watches. Put jangly keys and other personal pocket essentials in your kit bag.

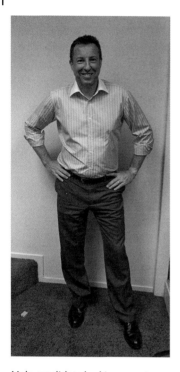

Male candidate looking smart

Advice for Women

- **Skirt or trouser suits** are popular. Tailored dresses look great but make sure you can move well. Lots of women don't wear jackets. Go for tailored and simple.
- Consider a **knit top** rather than blouse – you don't want to flash the patient when you bend over and you don't want any buttons to come undone accidentally, and have to hold your shirt together with Neurotips.
- Make sure your **skirt** sits on the knee or below, and you can sit and kneel comfortably.
- **Trousers** – same rule for nicely fitted, well-hemmed trousers as the males. Too tight and you run the risk of ripping out the

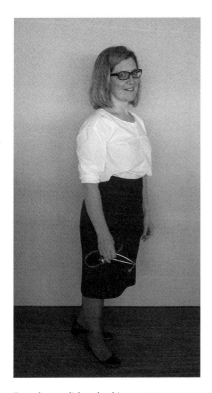

Female candidate looking smart

crotch seam when eliciting an ankle jerk. Too loose just looks sloppy.

- Get a **haircut** the week before. Make sure hair is clean and washed. If you have long hair, tie it neatly back.
- Keep **jewellery** simple. No dangly earrings or jingly bracelets.
- Subtle **make-up and perfume** – don't set off the patient's asthma.
- **Short nails** free of nail polish.
- Make sure your shoes are smart, polished, clean and worn in. Avoid very high heels – stumble around in your Jimmy Choos at the celebration dinner.

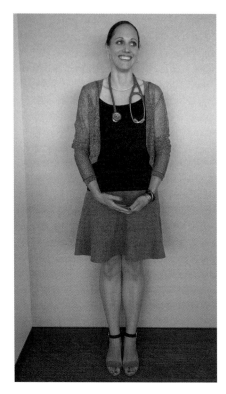

Female candidate wearing a … less than suitable outfit

Paeds Point

All the above advice is true for you too, but even more so. In your outfit, you need to be able to chase a toddler under a table, in front of a parent and three examiners, with your dignity intact, underwear invisible and seams robust. No mean feat.

- **Women** – a short tight dress will look ridiculous if you are chasing around after twins in your developmental short case. High heels – you could squash small fingers, and howling from the room during a long case seldom bodes well. When trying on your outfit, you need to be able to commando-crawl along the fitting room floor with ease.
- **Men** – a fashionable pale grey fitted slimline suit will look dapper on the streets of Melbourne. If you put this to the test of a cheeky child with a packet of Twisties, you will end up with visible boxer shorts as the seams rip while you sit in the chair. The suspicious orange fingerprints all over the jacket collar will destroy the shred of credibility that remains. When selecting your suit, make sure you can do jumping-jacks and touch your toes.

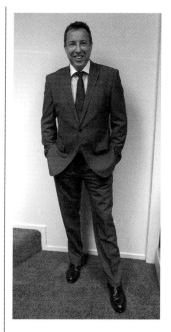

Before: Male candidate looking dapper … for now

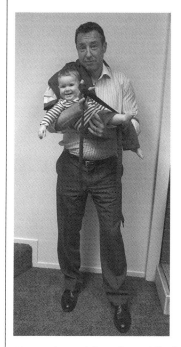

After: Male candidate after a difficult short case

The 'Infection Control' Effect

We are in no doubt that infection control will make its mark on the exam, as in the UK. This may be in the form of banning ties, ensuring everyone is bare below the elbows and compulsory 30-second hand washing or hand gel. We strongly suggest following usual protocols of alcohol gel before and after patient contact in the exam, just like you would do at work. There is minimal time to present in a short case, so a full 30 seconds hand-wash would take too long.

Summary

- The two weeks of ground work before you go anywhere near a patient are crucial. Make sure you take this time to rest, change your mindset and get organised.
- To pass on the day, you need at least two out of three of the following: being a good doctor, luck on Exam Day and to have put in the practice. Three out of three is best.
- Everyone has to ask for help for the Clinical Exam. Get humble.
- If you work in a hospital with no organised teaching sessions, you have your work cut out, but you can still prepare adequately and go on to pass. Get other candidates in your region on board. Seek out local experts and those further afield to help fill in gaps.
- Buy the books.
- Register and book in early to preparation courses.
- Get your kit bag together, or borrow one from a previous candidate.
- Start thinking about a smart yet practical outfit or two that you can wear for your upcoming practice sessions, and on Exam Day.
- Personal hygiene is very important.

14

How to Start – Doing Your First Practice Cases

Two weeks have passed, you have assembled your kit bag, have shopped for new clothes and feel like a bit of a Charlie standing there in your snazzy outfit. Now all you have to do is practise. Find a way of collecting and sharing (in a confidential way) details of inpatients who give a good history or have good signs and don't mind people practising on them. Most patients are quite chuffed to be asked, especially if they are waiting for rehab or a valve replacement. Sometimes a practice examiner will give you names of suitable long cases; other times you need to find your own. If you are at a small hospital, you will need to plan field trips to bigger hospitals with subspecialties to get a good breadth of cases.

There are a few legends out there who managed to be in the hospital for 120 days straight pre-exam. The rest of us managed 2–3 evenings after work, a half-day one weekend, and spent the rest of the weekend recovering and reading.

Your weekly clinical exam timetable might look something like this:

Mon	Tues	Wed	Thurs	Fri	Sat	Sun
Organised short case teaching		On-call day		Long case at lunch-time	3 h of short case practice	2 or 3 h book work. Type up long cases
	2 h of short case practice after work with study group		2 h of short case practice after work	Long case review	1 h book work	Collapsing in a heap

How to Pass the RACP Written and Clinical Exams: The Insider's Guide, Second Edition. Zoë Raos and Cheryl Johnson. © 2017 John Wiley & Sons Ltd. Published 2017 by John Wiley & Sons Ltd.

It is really hard to practise for the Clinical Exam. Each practice short case takes at least 45 minutes when you start. Long cases are invariably interrupted, never start on time and it can be quite a challenge finding your practice examiner afterwards.

Know Your Enemies

Know them well. It is by knowing your enemies that you can overcome them.

- Mealtimes and visitors
- Ward rounds
- Medication time
- Nap time
- Missing notes
- Patients away having an investigation/physiotherapy
- Sick patients – it is rather common for pre-exam registrars to sort out acute medical problems

A Few Tricks of the Trade

- For short cases, send your most charming study groupie to ask the patient nicely.
- Explain that you are experienced doctors studying to be specialists.
- Thank the patient before and afterwards.
- Making the patient a cup of tea (as long as not NBM) is a nice touch.
- If they say no, leave them alone. Tell others to leave them alone too.
- Weekend mornings (before the onslaught of visitors) are the optimal time for study group short cases with less competition for the patient's time. Long cases and organised sessions have to fit in with your practice examiners.

Practising Cases – Who Can Help You the Most?

All sorts of people will help you pass. Family members, patients, the helpful shop assistant in the suit shop, your study group, your beloved boss from three years ago … it is impossible to pass the Clinical alone.

One of the biggest helps (that, of course, is the most difficult to ask for) is to get practice examiners to supervise short cases (then grill you afterwards) and long case presentations (also followed by a good grilling).

Who Can Help Me Pass This Exam?

Examiners

The best people to practise any case with are examiners. You will very quickly get an idea of the standard required to pass – either an uplifting or deflating experience. Candidates realise too late and en masse that doing a long or short case with an examiner is gold. Be organised, find out the current or previous College examiners in your region and ask for practice sessions with these popular people months before the exam.

Consultants

Consultants are great for supervising both short and long cases. Some consultants are more constructive than others, so ask around. Don't be afraid to do cases with 'mean consultants', it is far better to have a grilling in a practice case than fall to pieces on the day. You will know a surprising number of consultants in your hospital. A good strategy is to email them individually with flexible times and dates for practice cases. Teeing up patients with signs and observing short cases takes up a lot more time than sending you off for a long case. Another excellent strategy, especially if there is a subspecialty you've never done and don't know a lot about, is to arrange to tag along to a specialty outpatient clinic for a morning or afternoon. This is a great opportunity to see clinical signs, get some teaching and get a feel for the particular psychosocial challenges in that area of medicine.

Senior Registrars

Senior registrars are better than your study buddies for short and, especially, long cases. These people have been through the exam and have a realistic idea of the standard required. They may be subspecialty registrars and have a little cache of patients with fantastic signs to show you. It is often a good idea to start your practice cases with senior registrars to get an idea about how to structure both a short and a long case.

Other Useful People to Get to Know

Anyone who has passed the British MRCP exam is great. The Brits are fantastic at the psychological art of putting on a show, looking slick, saying the right things at the right time. This is really handy for short case practice.

Your Study Group

Study group formed the lion's share of our short case preparation. Examining a patient in front of your peers, while nerve wracking, hones your confidence, skills and clinical acumen. It was useful to do short cases with different people. We learnt all sorts of little tricks and useful phrases and ironed out bad habits.

Once you've each got about five properly supervised long cases under your belt and have critically appraised them yourself, get the study group together over pizza and re-present the cases. You will learn from each other only with experience for long cases. We weren't specific and constructive enough to provide decent feedback at the start.

Yourself

There is very little point in sneaking around the hospital alone, trying to elicit signs for short cases, or doing long case presentations alone without a supervisor to grill you first. It is only by practising in front of others, with all that risk of humiliation, that your skills will improve at a fast enough pace to get you ready for Exam Day. It is useful to repeat your long case presentations to yourself the evening after, even recording your presentation and listening back (shudder), and to practise your short case discussion routines in front of the mirror.

Family Members, Partners or Anyone Non-Medical

Attack these healthy volunteers with your tendon hammer and stethoscope while you hone your short case routine. Non-medics can give good general advice on reducing 'ahs' and 'ums' but don't have the knowledge to grill you properly or spot a nasty mistake in your summary or presentation.

It is very good practice for you to supervise juniors doing cases, as this helps you to get into the examiner's shoes. It is not really useful to do short cases with the students as examiners, as they won't be mean enough.

Mock Exams: Well Worth the Humiliation

If your hospital or one nearby has a Clinical mock exam, sign up. You don't have to trawl around for patients or someone to examine you, it's under exam conditions, and outpatients are brought in specially – a completely different group to most inpatients, more well with chronic problems, less acute problems and resemble patients you are going to get on the day.

Some candidates feel too scared to attend the mock exam with all the attendant scrutiny and criticism. Gird your loins, be brave and turn up! If you fail miserably, it will feel awful but in this exam the harshest lessons are the most necessary. We all made a series of terrible stuff-ups in the mock exam. We licked our wounds and learned a lot. The mock exam is good practice for moving on after a bad case and learning how to keep your cool.

Summary

- Be organised. Work out who in your hospital and beyond will be useful to help with short and long cases and contact them early to book in cases over the next three months.
- Think about specific gaps in your clinical experience and proactively bridge them by arranging cases, or attending a half-day clinic in that specialty.
- Examiners, consultants and senior registrars are the best supervisors for long cases.
- Most short case preparation is done in study groups with some supervised sessions.
- If your centre is not well organised for teaching, you (and any other candidates in your area) will need to organise all your own teaching – difficult but not impossible.
- Sign up for any mock exams you can.

15

An Introduction to the Long Case

What is a Long Case Anyway?

A long case is where you are given 60 minutes with a patient in which to:

- take a history
- examine the patient
- construct a differential diagnosis
- formulate a problem list based on your findings
- prioritise and interpret investigations
- show the examiners that you are a sound clinician, with a good attitude and a sensible approach to clinical problems.

You are then given 10 minutes preparation time sitting by yourself in a cold and lonely corridor, perhaps with a bulldog* or time-keeper giving you funny looks. After this, you enter a room with two examiners and present your case for around 10–12 minutes. Your case presentation is followed by about 13–15 minutes of 'question and answer time' with the examiners.

60 min	10 min	10–12 min	13–15 min
Time in room with patient to take history, examine and start organising the presentation	Case prep outside the room	Present case to examiners	Grilling from examiners

*The College does not employ actual canine bulldogs; rather, bulldogs are registrars who assist on the day.

How to Pass the RACP Written and Clinical Exams: The Insider's Guide,
Second Edition. Zoë Raos and Cheryl Johnson.
© 2017 John Wiley & Sons Ltd. Published 2017 by John Wiley & Sons Ltd.

The long case marking schedule

The mark	History	Examination	Synthesis	Insight	Management
1	No structure to history. Superficial with details	No structure to examination	Most issues not identified or prioritised	No attempt to recognise impact of disease	Unable to interpret investigations. Unable to formulate management plan
2	Poorly presented history. Missed out key points. Disorganised	Missed significant physical signs	Needed a lot of prompting to establish a problem list	Didn't recognise most aspects of the disease and impact on patient and family. Didn't take life-lines	Difficulty interpreting investigations and poor management plan
3	Left out key parts of history	Missed some important physical signs but found others	Poor prioritisation of problems. Had a problem list, but not prioritised in the right order.	Didn't recognise all aspects of the disease and its impact on patient and family	Errors interpreting investigations. Disorganised approach to requesting investigations. Management plan lacks confidence
4	Complete history	Found all the signs	Thorough and prioritised problem list	Understands impact of disease (physical and psychological) as well as effect the treatment and prognosis have on patient and family	Appropriate interpretation of investigation results. Sensible and balanced approach. Recognises adverse effects of treatment
5	Complete history with emphasis on most important aspects	Found all the signs plus relative negatives	Thorough problem list divided into more important and less important issues	Empathetically explores subtle issues impacting on patient and family	Thorough and appropriate management plan with insight into impact of the disease
6	Complete history with empathetic extraction of the 'hidden gold'	Finds all the signs plus subtle signs that support diagnoses	Finds all major and minor problems, carefully PRIORITISED	Maturely conveys subtle and difficult aspects of functioning. Demonstrates balance and sophistication with social support	Thorough management plan with discussion of long-term impact
7	Exceptional history. The detail! The pithy summaries! The seamless flow! The emphasis on key points!	Perfect examination. Utterly perfect	Excellent problem list with understanding of how problems interact, like a complex game of chess	Complete, thorough understanding of psychological and social aspects along with everything else	Excellent management plan including all of the above, plus discussion of prognosis if appropriate

The font is small but the importance of this table is great. 4/7 = Pass. Deploying the examiner's benefit of the doubt can add another half-mark (see page 78). Annoying the examiner when you've otherwise done a good job can dock a half-mark. Most candidates grovel around the 3s for the first few practice long cases. This is soul destroying, but a crucial part of learning what a 4 feels like. In order to know what it feels like to nail a long case, you must first know what it is like to completely stuff some up. Please note that lots of the categories in this marking schedule include words like organised, confident, structure and prioritised. These are all skills that can be learnt.

Point to Prove in the Long Case

In an ideal world, our patients would come to clinic on time, know why they were there and know all their medications by heart. They would listen carefully to our advice and then go home to religiously take their tablets/dialyse three times a week/adopt a graduated exercise programme. They would thank you for your efforts, bake you some ANZAC cookies and send you a card at Christmas.

The College knows that this is a complete fantasy. They have developed the long case as a test of how well you perform in the real world. The long case is about real people with social issues, incredible disabilities and complex inter-related medical problems. The patients selected are nice enough to give up a day of their lives so you can (hopefully!) demonstrate to the College that you are a confident, competent practitioner of medicine who deserves to progress to advanced training.

To make the exam fair, the examiners are blinded to the case, just like you. Both examiners have 40 minutes with the patient – 20 minutes to take a history and 20 minutes for examination. They collect their thoughts as a duo, are given an envelope of relevant investigations for that patient along with a brief problem list and decide on the crucial parts of the history, examination and prioritised problem list against which the candidate is assessed.

Aspects of a Long Case

It is hard to explain, let alone do, a long case if you've never seen one presented before. Ask your Director of Physician Training if a mock long case could be presented by a consultant or senior registrar to get you all on the right track. If nothing like this can be organised, read our templates, book in a practice case with a sympathetic examiner and give it your best shot. The consultant or registrar examining your first practice case will soon give you some pointers to get it together.

There are five areas that get you brownie points in the long case. The emphasis is on keeping things simple, logical and safe. The standard you are expected to achieve is that of a registrar at the end of their basic training, not a subspecialist. You will be forgiven for not knowing what the chemotherapy is for T-cell lymphoma. You won't be forgiven if you forget to ask if the patient needs home help or not.

1 Take a history and ask relevant questions

- You ask asthma patients if they smoke, what triggers their asthma, how many pets, number of admissions to ICU, what medications work and get a family history of atopy (brownie point).
- Or ... you just list 'asthma' as a problem (disappointed sigh).

Look at the marking schedule for what is expected for a history to pass. Your history presentation needs to be complete and accurate, presented in a timely fashion and require minimal requests for clarification from the examiners.

2 Examine a patient in a relevant way

- You measure your diabetic patient's lying and standing BP as well as examining him for sensory neuropathy and performed fundoscopy (gold star).
- Or ... you mention that your diabetic patient didn't have clubbing or HPOA (huh?).

The marking schedule states you need to find all the signs. There are more marks for finding subtle and important negatives, and more again for a highly organised presentation of complex findings.

3 Know about psychosocial issues and how they influence the patient and their life

- You talk about the patient not taking his medications because he can't afford to pay for his prescription since he lost his job as a bus driver after being declared medically unfit to drive (beautiful!).
- Or ... you talk about bad BSLs because the patient doesn't take medicines (not bad).
- Or ... you talk about poorly controlled BSLs (boring).

There is a whole section in the marking schedule on the impact of illness on the patient and family. To pass, you must convey to the examiners that you understand how this particular patient's physical and psychological function is affected. This needs to come through not just in the social history but also be painted through the entire history.

4 List and prioritise multiple problems

- Do you crumble and fumble because the patient has a kidney transplant *and* hypertension *and* diabetes (yawn).
- Or can you list them all and then talk about the second two problems being exacerbated by the first (pretty good)?
- Or can you discuss them all, but emphasise that a gouty toe is actually the patient's biggest problem as it is stopping him from going to a bowls tournie (jackpot!)?

Synthesis and priorities is another whole marking column. You pass this section if you identify all the major problems, and get them in the correct order. This is why we recommend giving yourself extra time in the room, as takes a wee while to work out what is the crucial problem, what is the biggest concern to the patient, what is the biggest problem to the carer/parent/spouse if present, and what is the most pressing medical problem needing urgent attention.

5 Have a sensible, orderly approach to investigating and managing each problem

- 'I would manage Mr F's severe, predominantly left-sided heart failure by reviewing investigations to date for the underlying cause, looking at exacerbating factors, and use both non-pharmacological and pharmacological approaches to treating his symptoms and improving his prognosis. I would involve Mr F's family, a Pacific Support worker together with his GP to get a coherent management plan to improve compliance and understanding' (thank you, well done).
- 'I'd call a cardiologist and get an ICD' (missed the point).

Look at the marking schedule. To pass this section, examiners want you to have a plan that is appropriate, sensible and balanced. They want you to describe side effects and harm from treatments. You may also tick off more marks for impact of illness.

There is a knack to passing a long case, and a real art to nailing one. The knack can be learned with understanding and practice. The College knows from all your assessments that you can take a good history, examine a patient accurately, make a diagnosis and get a management plan together. What turns everyday occurrences into a long case is how the information is taken, organised, presented and discussed. You need systems for collecting the information, prioritising it all and being able to discuss it. You need to control your nerves so that all the skills you've gained every day at work are not thrown out the window when faced with a tricky case.

Practising for Long Cases

A Long Case – 95 Minutes

Let us begin with our old foe – the clock. Sixty minutes with one patient. Ninety-five minutes from start to finish, including a bit of a grilling. Seems like loads of time. It isn't. One of the biggest challenges to Clinical Exam candidates is getting your timing right for the long case. You will get faster at keeping to time with practice.

How to use your 95 minutes effectively in practice and on Exam Day

Time with the patient: **60 minutes**	**1 minute apologising in advance** – apologise to the patient for rushing them and (to all intents and purposes) interrogating them. Emphasise this is a big day for you. Ask them to help you pass the exam by telling you what they told to the examiners. Spend 15 seconds sorting out your notes (numbering cards, dividing up your piece of paper).
	25 minutes on history – 'the open-ended question has no place in the long case'. It takes practice to get good at taking a variety of histories, and getting yourself and the patient through a lot of questions in very little time.
	15 minutes on examining (all the while continuing to fill gaps in your history) – this has to be a pretty thorough but relevant examination, including cranial nerves, upper limbs, lower limbs, thyroid and any relevant joints. Examiners love finding a sign that you missed!

	20 minutes (yes, 20 whole minutes) writing up your presentation in the room, asking the patient all the questions you missed out in the history or having another look at physical signs ('I forgot to ask if you smoked').
	1 minute – after the knock on the door (or your alarm goes off), thank the patient sincerely for participating, and check with them there's nothing you've missed.
	Paeds Point: for adolescents, you will need to allow for time alone with the young person.
Time outside the room: **10 minutes**	Write your opening gambit and closing statements. Write your discussion table. Look over your notes. Say the key parts out loud to yourself a few times.
Time with the examiners:	**10–12 minutes** — **Case presentation** – it should take around 10 minutes to get through your opening gambit, history, exam, summary statement and problem list. Examiners can jump in a bit early.
	12–15 minutes — **Grilling session** (**question and answer time**) – the length and format are variable in practice cases and also on Exam Day. The examiners may let you talk non-stop about your management plan or interrupt every five seconds with questions. This is *not* a reflection of your performance but a reflection of the examiner's style. Be prepared for anything.

How Many Long Cases Should You Do?

Some candidates have an uncanny ability to see through the pitfalls and get to the crux of the issue. The rest of us need to know which questions to ask beforehand and have a template for common conditions. Some of us did 20 cases because we had cruisy jobs, too much time on our hands and were terrified of failure. Other slick first-time candidates did three long cases in total! The key is to start early and do enough cases so that you understand the whole long case style of presentation. Ensure you can stick to the allotted time, organise the case and present it confidently. At least one long case a week is about right.

If you've done seven cases and you're still struggling to achieve 4s, it's time to stop and take stock. Talk to a trusted consultant about where you might be going wrong. Go back to basics and try taking the time limit off for a couple of cases so you get to know what a passing case is like. A night spent writing up your cases perfectly at home and presenting them again to a supportive and helpful senior is time well spent. Have a look at Chapter 30, How to Fail, which has excellent tips on overcoming nerves and improving presentation skills.

Practicalities of Practising

Present your practice long cases to your long-suffering consultants and post-exam registrars.

- Book in a time for the long case that suits you and your practice examiner. Know when you will be starting the case, what time you will be meeting your examiner and where.
- Some consultants will find a 'good case' with lots of history and social stuff to discover. Other consultants will expect you to find a case yourself.
- A back-up case is always a good idea in case the first patient is called away to an investigation, has a visitor or is off the ward.
- Once you've got a few cases under your belt, ask your supervisors for specific cases to plug knowledge gaps.

Tee up the practice case so that it is under exam conditions as much as possible. What we mean is:

- the patient knows ahead of time that you're coming to see them and why
- you know nothing about the patient
- you have a list of their current medications but do not have access to their clinical notes
- you won't be interrupted
- you keep to time
- you give yourself the 10 minutes at the end sitting somewhere uncomfortable to prepare the case
- you aim to present the case to the 'examiner' straight away (so that you really do only have 10 minutes 'thinking time', not one week mulling it over).

Try to **present the case under exam conditions**. This involves a 10–12-minute presentation followed by 13–15 minutes of question time. It will be hellish, but avoiding a grilling will get you nowhere.

Ask for **feedback** and improvement tips. Be warned that there is always room for improvement, and everyone's a critic. Give a copy of the marking schedule to your examiner. See Chapter 31 for more advice on providing constructive feedback.

After the case, go home and **rewrite the presentation again**, making it better and adding in areas you missed. Present to yourself or your study group. Rewriting and perfecting your long cases is some of the most valuable prep work you can possibly do for this exam. Save your notes so you can refine your presentation style as the weeks go by and review them again in the week of the exam.

Watch other candidates present cases (and let them watch you). It's not as daunting as you think and you pick up lots of useful tips from each other.

Stick to your presentation style (once you have found one that works!) as it makes your presentations consistent, organised and calm. This is quite difficult, as every practice examiner will have his or her method that will be different from yours. Change your style if the suggestion makes sense, especially if you get consistent feedback over two or three long cases that a change in presentation style or format is needed. The next chapter has more specific advice about style.

Don't book any cases in the final week; a bad case will put you off your game.

What to Do If There Aren't Enough Patients to See

Don't despair because there's been no case of SLE at Taranaki Base Hospital for the past month. Consider working out a template and using it for imaginary patients. For example, imagine the crumbliest renal failure or rheumatoid arthritis patient you can, then work out a template of what issues need to be covered. Work out what rapid-fire questions you would ask your imaginary patient (where they dialyse/ how often/transplant list, etc.) and consider what issues might come up on that patient's problem list.

Thinking through the management issues of imaginary patients is more valuable (and time efficient) than seeing an extra 10 cases of the same old airways disease or heart failure that you already know how to do.

Key Long Cases

There are patients who seem get dragged in for the exam year after year. The contents page of Talley and O'Connor lists most types of long cases that crop up. If you are completely over the top, you might try and do a practice case of every one of these patients before the exam. Be warned – this strategy may lead to you completely freaking out.

For cases you don't see in real life, use your imagination. Work out what key questions you would ask the patient, how a problem list could look and essential management strategies for each problem. Here are a few 'old favourites' we came up with:

- Diabetic patient with complications
- Renal patient:
  - approaching dialysis
  - on dialysis
  - renal transplant
- Rheumatoid arthritis with complications
- Scleroderma
- SLE
- Neurodegenerative conditions:
  - multiple sclerosis
  - motor neurone disease
  - Parkinson's disease
- Epilepsy with management issues or pregnancy
- HIV
- IHD with complications
- Congestive heart failure
- Asthma/COPD/cystic fibrosis/bronchiectasis
- Transplant
- Liver disease
- Inflammatory bowel disease with complications

Paeds Point

Just like your adult medicine colleagues, you need to be prepared for anything. The common long cases that you must master include:

- Cerebral palsy/complex disability
- Epilepsy (usually combined with other conditions)
- CF and complications
- Oncology (usually in remission)
- Spina bifida
- CHD
- Developmental delay
- ADHD and learning difficulties
- Any of the above involving an adolescent in transition to adult medicine.

The contents page of *Examination Paediatrics* will guide you towards any deficits in your knowledge base

Taking Orderly Notes for Your Long Case

There are many ways of taking notes in a long case. Once you choose an option that works, stick to it. It is OK to practise your first few long cases with prewritten templates, but get out of this habit. On the day, any written material is total contraband. Your notes will not be handed in to the examiners for marking. If you try and write down everything (just like when clerking a patient), you will run out of time. Use key words that will prompt you. For example, '30 cigs' may be all that is needed to remind you to talk about how much they smoke, how long they have smoked, attempts at quitting in the past. Use your notes as an *aide-mémoire*.

It's also helpful to jot down reminders for things to check in the examination while taking the history. For example, if the patient mentions they have an AV fistula for dialysis or have symptoms of peripheral neuropathy, write those down to remind yourself to examine this area carefully.

Cards

Supporters will point out the nice subtle nature of a stack of A6 cards. They make you feel like you are giving a speech and encourage eye contact with the examiners. Cards can be your best friend when you have a waffly or complicated patient. When the patient jumps between diabetes, immunosuppression, the failed renal transplant and their abusive spouse, you can write each problem on a new card, then get back into the driving seat for the history once the main problems have been disclosed.

As well as a card per problem, you will need a SHx/FHx card, a medication card, an examination card and one card for the opening gambit and the summary. You will then need a card with your discussion table.

There are some warnings.

- Make sure you don't have too many cards. One card per minute of speaking is plenty, that's about 10–12 cards maximum.
- Number your cards in case you drop them, and use a small bulldog clip.

A4 Paper and Folders

This works well if you are a 'mind-map' person and find that cards aren't big enough.

- A4 photocopy paper works well. Avoid shuffling ultra-thin paper – it's distracting.
- Limit the number of pieces of paper you use or you will just look like you are using giant cards. You should only need about three sides of paper.

One method is to have an A4 folder or clipboard that contains two pieces of A4. All you need to do is open the folder like a book and turn each piece of paper once during the presentation.

Many candidates use an actual manilla folder to write on, with specific areas to document their notes. The only danger with folders is that small candidates tend to hide behind them, and can appear tiny and terrified.

Everyone needs a scrap piece of paper for jotting things down in passing. That way, you don't have to interrupt the patient all the time, and can go back and ask about that 'kidney problem you mentioned'.

Whatever option you choose, take your own supplies on the day. Clipboards and paper are available, but it is comforting to use your own stuff. Highlighters or coloured pens are helpful as prompts to points that you want to emphasise while you are speaking.

Role of the Study Group for the Long Case

Just because the Clinical Exam is an individual exam, it doesn't mean that the study group should be abandoned. After studying together for the last year or so, you may all get withdrawal! Study groups are great places to discuss cases, present cases to each other and work on management plans for particular problems. We all tackle a problem differently and a collaborative approach will help you prepare well.

Many groups will present their long cases of the week to each other, provoking constructive debate about better ways to summarise and manage all the problems. It is only possible for this to be a constructive and critical exercise once you've all done about five long cases. You can also divide up those tricky topics that often come up and need a few hours to sort out. Some examples:

- management of the recalcitrant smoker
- management of the socially isolated patient

- management of the poorly compliant patient
- management of a patient with transport issues
- management of the alcohol-dependent patient
- management of a patient with financial issues.

Summary

- The long case is a test of how you cope in the real world with real patients.
- There are 95 minutes from the very start to the very end of a long case. Timing is absolutely crucial.
- Develop a system for taking brief but organised notes for your long cases.
- Plan to do at least one long case per week in the lead-up. Some candidates need to do more and others less, but about 12 practice cases works for most.
- Get accurate feedback from your practice examiners by giving them a copy of the marking schedule and asking for advice on how to improve your performance – more on this shortly.
- Learn to critically appraise your own long cases.
- Your study group is a great way to workshop long cases even more, and figure out how to squeeze out even more marks.

16

Mastering and Presenting your Long Case

Now you know a little about long cases – what they are and how they are marked. To get the marks, you need to ask the right questions and discover all the issues – missing a kidney transplant is irretrievable.

Conversely, you won't get points if your presentation is waffly and you don't tell the examiners what you discovered. You may have taken an excellent history and have a really good understanding of all the issues but if you don't *sound* that way, the examiners assume that you are struggling and mark you down.

Your opening gambit needs to hit the examiners like a refreshing splash of water. There is absolutely no place for a 'big reveal' at the end of the long case. Immediately tell them what the major problems are. The examiners then know you have a good handle on the case right from the start. You are well on the way to passing, perhaps nailing, your long case.

A Suggested Style for Long Case Presentation

We quickly lost the medical student style of presentation. It takes too long, weighs heavily on an examiner hanging off your every word, leaves all the important information until the end and doesn't quickly show the examiners that you are aware of the major issues. Anyway, long cases often have no presenting complaint – they tend to be outpatients with stable problems, brought in especially for the exam.

How to Pass the RACP Written and Clinical Exams: The Insider's Guide,
Second Edition. Zoë Raos and Cheryl Johnson.
© 2017 John Wiley & Sons Ltd. Published 2017 by John Wiley & Sons Ltd.

Medical student style	FRACP style
Presenting complaint	Opening gambit, there often is no presenting complaint
History of presenting complaint Past medical history	Medical problem list (encompassing each main problem and each part of the medical history in order of importance)
Medications	Medication history in fine detail, including allergies and over-the-counter drugs
Social history	Social history ++++, drugs, alcohol, smoking, finance when relevant, sexual history when relevant ...
Family history	Family history if relevant Family tree in paediatrics
Systems review	Relevant negatives only if necessary Developmental issues in paeds patients
On examination	Examination findings Observations, each system described in turn. Relevant positive and negative findings
Impression	Summary statement
Plan	Prioritised problem list
	Discussion of each problem in turn with an organised management plan taking into account the patient as an individual

> **Paeds Point**
>
> See below for special sections such as developmental milestones, education and other key things not to miss.

Organising Your Presentation

Knowing what a long case is, let alone coming up with an organised presentation, is a common problem for registrars. Review long cases and templates from other candidates, in this book and in textbooks (e.g. T&O and *Mastering the Medical Long Case*). Examine how the author divided up the case and organised the information into a coherent presentation. They are by no means the only formats for presenting, but they are worth having a look at if you haven't got your own style.

Work out which format you are going to use early on and then practise this way in every case you do. Changing the format of your presentation the week before the exam increases the chances of accidentally leaving out a section.

Some patients have a lot of problems. One of the skills you will be marked on is whether you can work out which parts of the history are important. Be succinct. Summary statements like 'macrovascular complications' and 'activities of daily living' help you impart maximum information with minimum words. It saves you time and stops the examiners getting lost in the details. It's akin to the difference between a patient giving a history of their problems and a good registrar summarising it for the postacute ward round.

Verbal Signposts

Make it obvious that there is a structure to your presentation. Use verbal signposts – a small pause, eye contact followed by 'in summary', 'in terms of social history', 'on examination' or 'this brings me to the problem list' as this reminds the examiners where the presentation is up to. You want them to feel like they are being lead down a well-trodden path rather thrashing blindly through the undergrowth. Verbal signposts make it easier on the examiners, particularly if you are the last long case of the day and your examiners are knackered.

Verbal signposts should also be used in the medical problem list. In a diabetic patient, a good signpost is 'in terms of control' or 'Mrs Brown's exercise tolerance is' in a patient with angina. These signposts allow the examiners to mentally 'tick off' aspects of your history to ensure it is comprehensive and complete.

Presenting a Case Well – Speech and Drama 101

There are many tips for presenting a case well. Most registrars are confident speakers at work and are skilled at summarising and synthesising, yet turn into blithering mumblers when presenting a long case. Deploy the skills you use every day at work when presenting patients on Exam Day. Speak clearly and convincingly. Speak with authority and confidence, with a big dose of humility and humbleness. Not too fast and not too slow. Make eye contact. There are smooth-talking, slick registrars who take to long cases like ducks to water, charming the examiners like a second-hand car dealer. The rest of us blathered, mumbled, frothed and fidgeted through our first month of practice sessions. We watched our practice examiners stare out the window in boredom, make slightly horrified looks as we guffed the social history and become increasingly exasperated as life-lines were ignored. This is the whole point of practising. We fail, we learn, we evaluate and we evolve so that we can pass on the day. It takes practice to develop a style that conveys your genuine concern, genuine interest and genuine enthusiasm. Chapter 30 has some excellent tips for candidates struggling with presentation skills.

Presentation Template That Worked for Us

Part 1: The Opening Gambit

- Includes demographic details and an overview of the patient's problems.
- Three sentences maximum; write it out and practise before going into the examiners.
- Make it short and snappy so the examiners think 'Wow, we are in for a treat here!' You just know when your opening gambit really sings.

Template

- **Who** is the patient (age/ethnicity/occupation or something interesting about them).
- **Why** they are here (an inpatient/an outpatient/brought in for the exam today).
- State **major** problem, list other problems in order of importance.
- Cite any **social** concerns (they always do).
- Currently, the problem from **Mr X's point of view** is … (whatever patient is most worried about).

Example of an effective opening gambit:

'I saw Mr X who is a 56-year-old Maori retired farmer. His major problem is poorly controlled diabetes with multiple microvascular and macrovascular complications. He also has chronic obstructive pulmonary disease precipitated by smoking, gout as well as multiple social concerns. Currently his main problem is his blindness and inability to drive.'

> **Paeds Point**
>
> 'I have seen Toby W with his mother, Sasha, for part of the time. Toby is a 14-year-old student from Palmerston North Boys High whose major medical problem is a failing live-donor renal transplant secondary to poor concordance with anti-rejection medication. He now faces dialysis. This is on a background of thin basement membrane disease and associated complications. There are significant social, educational and family stressors at play. Currently, Toby's major concern is his faltering relationship with his dad.'

Part 2: The Medical Problem List

- List each problem separately and talk about each one succinctly, including the relevant positives and negatives.
- Make sure you talk *most* about the major problems, and less for minor ones.

Each problem needs to be a summary. Hit the highlights and keep the fine details up your sleeve. This gives you something to talk about in the discussion. There isn't time in 10 minutes to parrot off the entire conversation. Part of the whole assessment of your presentation is how effectively the case is summarised and synthesised.

Possible Template to use for Each Major Problem

- **The name of the problem.** 'Mrs X's first problem is severe, polyarticular rheumatoid arthritis.'
- **When and how the diagnosis was made.** 'This was diagnosed 20 years ago after she presented with swollen hands to her GP, who carried out investigations and referred her to a private rheumatologist.'
- **List complications.** 'The disease is further complicated by extra-articular manifestations including pericardial effusions, Sjogren's syndrome and splenomegaly.'
- **Initial treatment.** 'Initially, Mrs X received gold injections. She was then changed to methotrexate…'
- **List treatments and associated complications.** 'She has received multiple courses of steroids, and was diagnosed with osteoporosis after a humerus fracture in 1995. Since then, she has taken bisphosphonate therapy.'
- **Current medications for the problem**. 'Currently she is on a tapering course of prednisone for a recent flare, with azathioprine as a steroid sparing agent.'

- **Functional limitations.** 'Despite extensive joint involvement, Mrs X works as a telephonist, mobilises with a walking stick and can drive a modified car.'
- **Monitoring and follow-up.** 'Mrs X's rheumatologist retired three years ago, and she's not found another. She sees her GP for repeat prescriptions and regular blood tests.'

For a **symptom** rather than a chronic condition, make sure you mention how long it's been present, associated symptoms, any relevant positives and negatives, current treatment and pending investigations. For example:

> 'Mr X's main problem is a three-month history of progressive exertional breathlessness which is associated with orthopnea, paroxysmal nocturnal dyspnoea and ankle swelling. Three months ago, he was able to walk the length of Brown's Bay beach but is now breathless walking to his letterbox. He denies cough, fever or sweating and has had no recent long-distance travel. Of relevance, he has recently changed his antihypertensives and stopped taking his diuretics.'

As you drift down the problem list, **use less and less detail** as this demonstrates to the examiner that you are aware that these problem exist but are not as important as earlier problems.

> 'Mr X's fifth problem is well controlled gout.'

This is a perfectly adequate statement and doesn't waste time.

Paeds Point

In amongst the problem list, you will need to include the following:

- Pregnancy
- Birth
- Neonatal history
- Development – milestones, presence or absence of delay, level of functioning, schooling

Sometimes, these will shoot straight to the top of the problem list itself. For example, in an autism spectrum disorder (ASD) case, development is the whole point. For congenital heart disease, the prenatal scans that diagnosed the tetralogy of Fallot and immediate neonatal history will be important parts of the discussion.

For more medical cases, the pregnancy, birth, neonatal history and development must be mentioned as important negatives after presentation of each problem to show the examiners that you have asked these questions.

Children with chronic health problems share many of the difficulties of children who don't have these, and carry a burden of concerns that other kids never face. It is important that you touch on the following when you take your history (with thanks to the RCH book).

- Sleep
- Hearing
- Eyes/vision
- Teeth/dentition
- Feeding/growth/nutrition
- Incontinence/toilet training
- Bones
- Puberty

Again, these will snuggle nicely into many problems, depending on the case. For the child with rheumatic heart disease, dentition will need a special highlight for endocarditis prophylaxis. For the child with Crohn's disease, nutrition and failure to thrive are especially important. For the young person with steroid-dependent juvenile arthritis, think of their bones. For developmental cases, you will check off incontinence. You need to think on your feet; the kid with ulcerative colitis might have horribly embarrassing incontinence, keeping him up all night, and he can't stay awake in class. The girl with severe autism might have toilet trained like a dream, sleep all night and be thriving at her special school, but mum is much more worried about early puberty and how she will manage menarche.

Part 3: Medication List

Some candidates are very adept at putting the medications throughout the medical problem list and this can work well … for some people. The inherent danger is that you miss out important medications and confuse examiners. For safety, we suggest mentioning key medications in the problem list and keep a proper section for all the pills and potions. Prepare a list of medications, which should be prioritised by importance and grouped by indication. The examiners may not require you to rattle off all the medications during the presentation. Other important pieces of medication history that need to be mentioned are:

- compliance/concordance. If the patient is non-complaint then what are the barriers to taking their medication?
- how the patient takes their medications – blister packs, bottles/boxes, dosette box
- allergies/intolerances
- OTCs
- vaccinations, particularly influenza and pneumococcal in the elderly or immune suppressed
- childhood vaccinations in paediatric case.

Many of these items seem trivial but the examiners expect you to mention them, or be able to answer questions during the grilling session.

Part 4: Social History

This is really, really important, where lots of marks come from and where you strike that 'hidden gold'. There are so many ways to present a social history that it is difficult to provide a template. You may incorporate parts of the social history into the problem list. You may find a mnemonic that helps you remember all the important bits. Your social history needs to be tailored to the individual patient and will be different depending on their age, cultural background and social connectedness. Many examiners are geriatricians who always take detailed social histories, so don't skimp! There is also an art to knowing what you don't need to include in a particular case.

Important aspects to consider in a social history include the following:

- **Employment history** – this is where you find the interesting things about your patient which can be used in your opening/closing statements. May be highly relevant for occupational health issues.
- **Family situation** – who do they live with? Do they have children? What are their social networks? Does their spouse/significant other have health issues that may impact on the patient? Are they caring for an unwell family member/spouse/significant other?
- **Home set-up** – this history needs to be tailored to the patient. A 40-year-old man who is mobile without assistance? Move your discussion to his antiretroviral medication regime. An 86-year-old

woman who relies on a low walking frame? Your time is well spent discussing stairs, rails, access to the property, access on/off bed and toilet, access into shower/bath and whether the patient has adaptive equipment. Also include whether the home is rented or owned.

- **Financial situation** – are they still working and does illness impact on their employment? Are they unemployed and wish to return to work? Are they on a benefit or the pension? Do they have adequate funds to pay for doctors/prescriptions/telephone, etc.?
- **Relationship with their doctors** – do they have a regular GP or do they see a different doctor in the practice each visit? This is important for continuity of care and can be one of the problems included in the problem list. Are they seen regularly within the hospital system?
- **Driving** – an older person who drives gives good insight into their functional capacity. If they don't drive then how do they get to the supermarket or to the doctor/hospital? Also think about how their medical conditions will impact on driving ability. Medical Aspects of Fitness to Drive is a really great resource and can be found at www.nzta.govt.nz.
- **Mobility** – do they need a mobility aid? Do *you* know the difference between a walking stick/quad stick/low walking frame/gutter frame/pulpit frame? If you don't, then ask your friendly physiotherapist. How far can they walk without stopping? What limits their mobility?
- **Activities of daily living** – are they able to shower/dress/toilet independently? Do they have personal care support for dressing/showering/meal preparation or do they rely on their spouse/significant other? Do they have housework assistance? Do they pay privately for a gardener or cleaner?
- **Cultural** – were they born in another country? Are they a refugee? Are they active within their cultural community? Do they want cultural support from the hospital?
- **Legal** – do they have an Enduring Power of Attorney? Have they made an Advance Care Plan? If you don't understand what these documents are, information can be found at www.justice.govt.nz or www.advancecareplanning.org.nz. Any Mental Health Act issues? Any Child Protection orders?
- **Sexual history** – can be awkward to bring up but is important, particularly impotence in a diabetic, activity tolerance in a patient with ischaemic heart disease/stroke, fertility issues in a young woman.

- **Tobacco/drugs/alcohol** – smoking history should be given in pack/years. Alcohol history is also important and should be considered in all patients regardless of age. Tailor substance and drug use to the individual patient.
- **Support agencies** – there are myriad disease-orientated charities and support agencies for adult and child patients (and their families), i.e. Parkinson's Society, Alzheimer's Association, Age Concern, the Cancer Society, CanTeen, etc. It's a good idea during your preparation to create a reference list with potential support groups.
- **Falls** – has your elderly patient had a fall within the last six months? This gives you a good indication of their functional ability and frailty.
- **Mood** – has their illness impacted on their mood?
- **Coping** – how are they managing at home with their illness? Are there improvements that can be made to allow them to cope better?
- **Memory** – have they had concerns about their memory?

We suggest turning to Chapter 21 for real-life long cases to see how the social history can be presented. It is very useful to have strategies up your sleeve for patients with multiple social problems when there is not time to review every detail in 60 minutes. Practical points for your discussion could include follow-up appointments, collateral history from family and GP, home visits and multi-disciplinary team review. This is a delicate balancing act in a long case, as outsourcing every problem to someone else is a cop-out and drives examiners batty.

Part 5: Family History

This is more important in some cases than others. A family history in an 84-year-old man with congestive heart failure is much less important than the 45 year old with Parkinson's disease. You may have already touched on this in the problem list if the medical condition has a familial inheritance. It is perfectly acceptable to use a one-liner such as 'There is no significant family history' if there truly isn't.

In paediatric and adult cases with a genetic flavour, a quickly drawn family tree can be a time-efficient way of capturing and presenting a complex family history.

Part 6: Systems Review

The systems review is a brillant catch-all to find out information that you may have missed during your 60 minutes with the patient to find hidden gold. If you find important information in the systems review, then include this in your medical history/problem list. It does not demonstrate good physicianly synthesis to include crucial information under a systems review in your discussion – leave that to the medical students. Hopefully, you will have touched on important negatives as you go. Essentially, this should be a one-liner: 'Nothing of note on systems review' because you've built all the juicy information from the systems review into your problem list.

Part 7: Examination Findings

Most examiners are used to hearing the examination findings grouped into one statement. Some candidates put the exam findings in the problem list. We do not recommend this. Present the exam findings as its own section after the history, in the traditional order.

- Description of the patient
- End of the bed-o-gram
- Observations
- Cardiovascular
- Respiratory
- Abdomen
- Neurological
- Special: functional/developmental/rheumatological etc.

Practise ways of summarising sections of the exam succinctly (e.g. 'pyramidal pattern of weakness in the left lower limb' or 'developmental milestones typical of a 2 year old') as it saves time and shows that you are putting the signs together. Include relevant negatives rather than report the absence of hundreds of irrelevant signs. It will save time and show that you were examining with a purpose. Short case practice is the best way to get slick at doing examinations, summarising your findings and presenting them succinctly.

Part 8: Summary Statement

This is where you finish reporting all the things you found and signal that you are in discussion mode. Pause, use a verbal signpost in a slightly louder summing up kind of voice.

'In summary... (short pause to alert dozing examiners) *Chrystal is a 17-year-old sickness beneficiary with severe, pan-enteric Crohn's disease. She has recently come off home parenteral nutrition after a prolonged hospitalisation following surgery for small bowel strictures and perianal disease. Chrystal has disclosed that she recently had unprotected sex whilst heavily intoxicated, which requires urgent review. She is also fearful of transitioning to adult services, is intermittently compliant with her adalimumab injections and has cellulitis over a new tattoo site.'*

Rather than rehashing your opening gambit, the summary statement shows the examiners that you have filtered through all the information and packaged up the key issues to prepare for ... brace yourself ...

Part 9: The Prioritised Problem List

It is *really* important to get this right. Remember how we keep saying that you will get marked on how well you can summarise the main issues? This is where the money is. Have another look at the marking schedule on page 112. Also, have a look at Chapter 21 where we have example long cases to see real-life problem lists in action.

- Make sure the examiners know the problem list is coming with a verbal signpost such as (pause) 'I have identified *x* number of problems, the first being...'.
- Include the problem of most importance to the patient. It can surprisingly be anything, from worries about dad losing his job, to moving house, to how long the kidney transplant will last this time, to not getting on with the GP. In the paeds exam, always identify the problem of most importance to the patient, *and also* the problem of most importance to the parent/carer.
- Issues such as bone protection, anticoagulation, multiple cardiovascular risk factors, social isolation can all be listed as individual problems, especially if you need more to talk about. Practise phrases that outline these problems succinctly.
- Make sure you have at least 5–8 real problems on the list that you can talk about, and that you have thought about how you will investigate, treat or potentially prevent each one.
- Another way of dividing up problems is whether they are *active* or *inactive*. First, list all active diagnostic, management and social issues. Then list inactive problems with less detail.

Part 10: Management Plan

This is the guts of the case and needs to flow nicely on from the problem list. This is where you demonstrate to the examiner how you will sort out each problem in an orderly way that makes sense. This is also where some keen examiners may start to grill you, throw curve balls and derail trains of thought.

We find the best way to handle the management plan is to draw up a discussion table as illustrated below. Examiners may want to jump the discussion straight to the third problem, and a table allows you to be flexible, keep in some control and reduce the fluster factor! Start drafting your discussion table during the hour with the patient and finalise it in your 10 minutes time in that cold, lonely corridor. Remember – you cannot possibly write all of this down during a real long case. There is not time. Use summaries and your own shorthand during the case itself. It is very useful after the practice long case is done and presented to retrospectively type the whole thing up.

Problem	Differential diagnosis	Investigations	Management plan
Presumed severe AS with SOB and syncope. Clinically has mixed valvular disease with TR and pHTN	CHF secondary to rate-related CM, ICM or other valvular disease	Bloods – Hb, renal function, BNP ECG Telemetry CXR Spirometry Echocardiogram Angiogram	Daily weight Salt and fluid restriction Diuretics Cautious use of ACEi Correct anaemia Discussion regarding surgery – AVR/TAVI Patient keen, but probably not an operative candidate
Management of falls risk	Exertional syncope secondary to severe AS Previous # and no bone protection Dabigatran	Bloods – coagulation screen Lying/standing BP monitoring ECG Telemetry Review CXR for undiagnosed osteoporotic #	Falls prevention strategies – hip protectors Bisphosphonate therapy Vitamin D Consider change to warfarin

(Continued)

(Continued)

Problem	Differential diagnosis	Investigations	Management plan
Social isolation	Depression Elder abuse	Depression score	Corroborative history with family and GP Refer to social worker Refer to Age Concern Arrange family meeting Encourage Mr P to get in touch with bowling club friends
Driving	Patient still drives. With syncope, not legal	All of above	Sensitive issue (social isolation) but obliged to inform LTSA Needs transport to appointments arranged Arrange transport to bowling club for social interaction

The Grilling

Every examiner (on the day and in the lead-up) will have a different approach to their 25 minutes with you. Most times you have 10–12 minutes to talk all the way to your problem list – the grilling and interruptions commence any time from this point. Some examiners don't say much and you need to keep talking for the whole 25 minutes. Other examiners will pounce as soon as the summary statement is finished, with verbal tussling needed to finish the problem list and start on the management plan. Your table is really useful, as it allows you to get back on track after an interruption and keep control of the discussion. In the example above, the examiner might have a detailed discussion with you about a spirometry finding. It is up to you to get the discussion moving forward to management of falls risk before the bell goes.

The Aftermath

At some point, the grilling will end. For practice cases, give your examiner a copy of the marking schedule at the start of your presentation and ask for honest (brutal) feedback. Some examiners go through the whole case blow by blow: where you passed, where you failed, how to get better, what you were wearing. Others say 'That was OK' and offer no constructive feedback. A copy of the marking schedule will help focus the discussion on areas that are progressing well and areas that need improvement. Have a look at Chapter 31 for giving and receiving constructive feedback.

We found it extremely useful to go home and rewrite the practice case, taking into account any feedback given by the practice examiner. We know that the last thing you feel like after doing a terrible practice long case is reliving the horror but this is the time that you learn the most. Drag out the textbooks and read around the cases and add parts that you had forgotten to do during the case. You won't forget twice!

After rewriting, each practice case should be filed away for later. Once you have done about five long cases, it is a very useful strategy to present your cases to your study group. Reviewing your long cases, and those of your colleagues, in the final weeks is excellent revision.

Sentences That Save Time and Sound Slick

Just like witty repartee, pithy summaries always pop in your head an hour after the case is done, so write them down and use them next time. Study group is great for brainstorming slick sentences. Here are some we came up with.

- 'Mr X has a number of macrovascular and microvascular complications of his diabetes, including end-stage renal failure, blindness, bilateral below-knee amputations and symptomatic, end-stage coronary artery disease.'
- 'Mrs W also has a number of complex social issues, but the most outstanding of these is pressure from her employer to take less sick leave.'
- 'Mrs F has had myriad admissions for neutropenic sepsis in the past three years.'
- 'Mr D describes many laparotomies relating to his Crohn's disease, his first at the age of 23.'
- 'Ms R has an array of issues revolving around the management of her HIV.'
- 'Master D and his parents struggle with the complex drug regime for his immune suppression.'
- 'Miss A has a good understanding of the complexities involved in managing her diabetes.'

- 'Although Mr G is most worried about access to increased home help, I have grave concerns about his non-intentional weight loss and a change in bowel habit.'
- 'Mr W's alcohol abuse has had a major effect on many aspects of life, aside from the heart transplant for cardiomyopathy.'
- 'I would like to start by talking about poor compliance, which I think is his biggest problem.'

Summary

- We recommend dropping the medical student style of presentation in favour of a problem-based approach.
- Carefully organise your presentation into clear parts. When presenting, use verbal signposts so that you take the examiners on the journey with you.
- It takes practice to be a slick long case presenter. Your first 4–5 cases will almost certainly be dismal … you will improve.
- Give practice examiners a marking schedule and ask for constructive feedback.
- When home, rewrite the long case as you would have done it in the ideal world with unlimited time. Re-present to yourself in the bathroom mirror and, later, to your study group. File it away for revision in the final week before the exam.
- You will learn slick sentences that summarise and save time. Write these down when you think of them.

17

Special Points for Paediatric Cases

 While we will continue to sprinkle Paeds Points throughout the rest of the book, this part deserved its own chapter. We also think adult medicine candidates could learn a lot from reading this chapter too – we certainly did – especially the bit about adolescents.

Specific Points About the Paediatric Long Case

Anticipate Boredom

Adult patients generally love nothing more than a sympathetic young physician trainee, hanging off their every word. Often parents and carers are the same. Child patients … not so much! It is surprising just how quickly a bored kid can rip a room apart. Anticipate boredom, and deploy tricks that not only keep the patient on your side but also assess aspects of the developmental exam. Ask the child to draw a picture or show off their hand-writing. Deploy a colouring-in book, a bouncy ball or a torch.

Brainstorm Common Childhood Problems and How to Solve Them

You need a practical approach to managing specific difficulties often encountered in childhood for all families. You need a little spiel for each of the common dilemmas of childhood, to show the examiners that you are a well-rounded trainee with an excellent understanding of general paediatrics. These spiels include:

- toilet training
- sleeping difficulties

How to Pass the RACP Written and Clinical Exams: The Insider's Guide, Second Edition. Zoë Raos and Cheryl Johnson.
© 2017 John Wiley & Sons Ltd. Published 2017 by John Wiley & Sons Ltd.

- tantrums
- fussy eating
- positive parenting programme for parental skills.

Forget-Me-Nots for Maximising Marks on Impact of Illness

Make sure you can demonstrate the impact of the illness or condition on the child, their family and community. Schooling, sports, after-school activities, sibling development, parental relationships and holidays all take a big hit with a sick or disabled kid in the family. Not only is it your job to identify these issues, but you must have sensible approaches to helping. Know about carer support, social workers, respite care and the role of all the other members of the multidisciplinary team. Know about transport support to get to clinic appointments, and have a good working understanding of Ministry of Health entitlements and benefits for children and their families.

Goals and Future Plans

These are really important for children and young people. For example, Tim, an able 17-year-old boy, is the front row forward in the first XV, but is heavily dependent on his mum for medication and clinic transport. He wants to go away to uni in two years. Talk about how transition of care is not just about doctors, but also about transitioning responsibility from mum to Tim. You will use Tim's goal of uni to engage him in the management of his ulcerative colitis.

Prognosis and Resuscitation Status

This is hard enough for physicians to talk about with adult patients. We take our hats off to our paediatric colleagues who care for dying children and their families. If handled sensitively, this is a way to demonstrate to the examiners that you understand that Millie, aged four, has inoperable congenital heart disease. She is getting sicker by the day. Her mum has an accurate understanding of the prognosis. Dad spends hours every night Googling possible cures and emailing international experts. In your discussion, outline how you would help guide the family through this difficult time, and help Millie achieve her goal of a first day at school and meeting a fairy.

Different Priorities for Different Members of the Family

You need to be able to focus on the main problem for the child *and* the main problem for the family. They are often different. For example, 15-year-old Scarlett's main problem is getting discharged home so she can go to the school ball with her boyfriend. Scarlett's dad is more worried about her impending acute rejection from her liver transplant. He might lose his job with all the time off travelling from rural WA to Perth for her multiple hospital visits. Both must be mentioned and are of crucial importance; if Scarlett self-discharges in defiance of her dad, she could end up very yellow very quickly!

Understand the effect of having a carer, grandparent or dad as the responsible adult rather than mum. Dad might play down the psychosocial aspects. Granny might be overly critical of the parents' ability to cope. A carer may have no idea what on earth is going on or be an amazingly engaged foster parent. You don't have to solve all the problems of the family (no one can), but emphasise that you would like to involve more family members to get a full picture of the situation, to improve the care of the child. It is acceptable to say that you get the sense that something else is going on that needs to be explored further, and give a clear plan about how you would do this.

Golden Words

Learn the following words and insert them into your presentation.

Reading these, there is much adult physicians can learn from paediatricians.

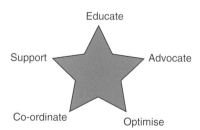

5 star words to use in a paediatric long case

The Developmental Case

This is an area where basic paediatric trainees have little exposure, but forms an important part of the Clinical Exam. Trainees are understandably terrified of developmental cases, as it is a subspecialty that is usually staffed by consultants and advanced trainees. You must put your fear aside. You can expect one developmental short case and possibly a long case on Exam Day, so it is well worth your while reading this section carefully and setting up specific developmental practice cases.

A Bit about Developmental Paediatrics

A developmental paediatrician uses standardised testing on a daily basis, but this is only a small part of the whole process. Developmental paediatricians get detailed referral letters from colleagues, assessments from SLTs and teachers and work within a multidisciplinary team. The children have extended appointments, in some cases spread over months, in order to reach a diagnosis. Paradoxically, it can be the more subtle difficulties that take the longest to label, whilst the barn-door diagnoses are less about the label and more about getting a support system built around a child and his or her family.

Developmental Paediatrics for Exam Candidates

It is impossible to replicate the full developmental assessment process in the exam, and the examiners know this. What is possible and achievable is a quick, less structured, and pragmatic assessment that a good general paediatrician would do before sending a referral to a developmental colleague. The developmental assessment is much more than ticking off a bunch of milestones against so-called norms. A ballpark idea of the child's developmental stage is gleaned. The strengths and difficulties of that child can be outlined. The immediate needs for the parents or carers can be established. Importantly, a plan involving the multidisciplinary team can be set under way. It is this less structured but highly useful assessment that comprises the developmental long case.

Milestones

Every paediatrics trainee needs to know their milestones for children aged six weeks, three months, six months, 12 months, 18 months, two years, 2.5 years, three years, four years and five years. Swot up on these. For school-aged children, add in cognitive function/academic progress with adaptive functioning/self-help skills.

Getting to Know the Basics of the Developmental Long Case

- **History** – this is where the money is. Take a detailed history from the parent and, if appropriate, the child.
- **Physical examination** – important, as there may be clues about a diagnosis, such as chromosomal abnormalities, dysmorphia or a neuromuscular condition. You need to be flexible in your physical examination to find/exclude all the appropriate signs.
- **Developmental examination** – see below.
- **Standardised assessments** – these are legion. Connor's Questionnaire for ADHD, the Autism Diagnostic Observation Scale, the WISC cognitive assessment, the SYSTEMS score for screening cognitive function in school-aged children and ABA for adaptive and functional assessment are but a few. A trainee is not expected to know these off by heart for the Clinical Exam. Demonstrating awareness and utility of these tools is expected to pass, with detailed knowledge for a higher mark. For example, in your management plan for a child with possible ADHD, you could say 'I would make an appointment with Sione and his family to complete a comprehensive assessment using the Connor's Questionnaire. This would add qualitative and quantitative information, and provides the multi-disciplinary team with information about areas of difficulty and also his strengths ...'.

There is a lot of ground to cover for a developmental case. Candidates quickly run out of time and get into a lather if they have a rigid checklist; 'First, need to assess gross motor. OK, vision next. Get out the vision chart. Now expressive language...' – this approach will take far too long. How then to fit in an entire developmental exam? The main tricks are as follows.

- Think on your feet.
- Adapt your exam (physical and developmental) based on the child's other presenting problems.
- Take full advantage of spontaneous displays.

Spontaneous Displays and How to Translate into 'Development-Speak'

Rosemary hasn't spoken a word during the exam despite temptation. She opens the zip on mum's handbag, finds some raisins, look at mum guiltily, mum says 'Oh, go on then', Rosemary opens the box, eats some then offers the box to you and mum.

- **Development-speak**: Fine motor and self-help skills appropriate for age. No expressive language exhibited, excellent receptive language, shared attention with mum and spontaneous social interaction with you, the examiner.

Daniel is reading a Spot book aloud with his mum chiming in and them both laughing. You see his cochlear implant across the room.

- **Development-speak**: Daniel has hearing difficulties, which are being assisted by his implant such that he has good receptive and expressive spoken language, at the level of a six year old.

You observe Manu hopping like a frog, saying 'reddit reddit' on the way to his dad for a hug.

- **Development-speak**: Gross motor, imaginative role-play and social interaction appropriate for a four year old.

Mum tries to tickle Stephan as he lines up the matchbox cars. He pushes her away and keeps on lining up the cars and looking at the wheels spinning.

- **Development-speak**: Repetitive play, fixed routine, difficulty with interruption, no shared attention despite mum intruding on play. Unable to assess receptive or expressive language.

How to Assess Domains Aside from Spontaneous Displays

Hopefully, you can see that the spontaneous display is your best friend. These can happen at any stage so make the most of them. As time is limited, you will need to open your 'bag of tricks' to bring out as many domains as you can. Use your powers of observation plus the right gear for the right developmental stage. After observing any spontaneous displays, add in some equipment to bring out what has not yet been demonstrated. You might give some blocks to a toddler, pencil and paper to a primary school child or a ball for anyone from three years upwards. There are some skills that cross into different domains, such as language and hearing, or social and language. This adds to the challenge of developmental assessment.

How to Describe What You Are Seeing

For the developmental short case, many candidates choose to talk as they go, explaining domains and milestones as they see them, then summarising at the end. This 'low road' is preferable to the 'high road' of saving it all up. You need to describe what you are seeing with qualitative abnormalities for each domain, comparing against norms for that age. Be careful in the language you use, be sensitive to the child and their carer. This is important for all paediatricians, but even more so in the exam. Use language like 'typically developing', 'atypically developing' and 'age-appropriate for...'. There is no place for the words 'normal' or 'abnormal' in the developmental exam. What is normal anyway?

Strengths and Difficulties

It is really useful to discuss the strengths and difficulties of your young patient, especially for the long case. Every child has strengths. By bringing these out, you demonstrate maturity and excellent powers of observation and you will have lots to talk about in your management plan.

> 'Sheena has marked global developmental delay across many domains. She has a warm and reciprocal relationship with her mum and dad. Sheena also has specific interests in Barbie dolls and enjoys watching *Home and Away*. I would work closely with the MDT to use these special interests to pique Sheena's interest and motivation. I would actively support her mum and dad as they are doing a great job, but are at risk of carer fatigue.'

Difficulties are obviously important too, and give you much to talk about in the discussion as long as you can come up with useful strategies.

> 'Rashid's trisomy 21, aside from physical complications including congenital heart disease, is strongly affecting his quality of life and that of his family through his behavioural difficulties. Rashid attending school is the most immediate priority. This

will maximise his educational potential and, importantly, help with the family dynamics. His parents are exhausted and disengaged with Rashid and his three older siblings.'

Just like in the adult long case, sometimes a difficulty is unsolvable. It is important, especially when gunning for high marks, to sensitively emphasise that there is no easy way out, and offer practical strategies.

'George's autism spectrum disorder is severe, with significant difficulties. His parents are motivated but exhausted carers. They have tried every therapy and are tuned in to all help available, in fact mum is the secretary of the Australian Autism Foundation and has trained as a therapist. George is failing to thrive physically because of limited dietary choices, has severe behavioural issues and does not sleep at night. It would be fair to say his family has tried everything. What would make the biggest difference here is increased family support and respite care in the first instance.'

Coming to a Conclusion in the Developmental Exam

Many candidates describe what they are seeing, but fail in the summary for both the short and long case. It is important that you practise coming to a conclusion in the developmental exam. For example:

'Thank you for asking me to assess Tom, a four-year-old boy, who I saw with his mother, Jillian. On developmental examination, his vision and hearing appeared grossly intact. He had the gross and fine motor skills expected at age two. Tom's language was age appropriate, but he was somewhat shy with less interaction expected socially for a four-year-old. Tom exhibited delayed self-help skills. In summary, Tom appears to have difficulties in the domains of language, social skills and gross and fine motor skills. My differential diagnosis includes...'

'Camille has many phenotypical features of Turner's syndrome. I focused on the developmental examination. Despite the many physical features of Turner's, Camille has reached and exceeded most developmental milestones expected for a five year old, including...'

Practice

The only way to get good at the developmental short case is (you guessed it) practice! An excellent source of subjects is the siblings of children stuck in hospital. They are often delighted to volunteer, the parents will be happy to have a semi-responsible adult look after their child for a while and everyone has a bit of fun. Practise on babies, toddlers and school-aged children. You will quickly remind yourself of the milestones, and how typically developing children present at certain ages. You will also appreciate the enormous breadth in what is typical, and gain confidence in summarising and the presenting style needed for this type of case. You will learn how to make the most of spontaneous displays. Use your study group, so that you can all learn from your successes and guffs.

For the developmental long case, ask around. Many children in hospital with physical illness will have concomitant developmental issues as well. Sometimes these poor kids are thoroughly bored, so playing with you, running around (or zooming in their wheelchairs) and drawing pictures is a relief. Make it fun for them. Your local general or developmental paediatrician will also have clinics where children undergo assessments, so ask if you can come along. You will learn a lot from seeing a slick developmental paediatrician in action, crawling on the floor, playing row your boat, pulling toys out of a bag like magic, throwing a ball, all whilst taking a history from the parent or carer.

The Adolescent Long Case

Adolescents scare the hell out of society, and out of many candidates. Try and change your mindset. There is so much to talk about! Young people are at the crossroads between childhood and adulthood. Their frontal lobe is totally out of whack with the rest of the brain, and this can make for chaos in life, and in the long case. Traditionally, adolescents turn up in the paediatrics exam, but there is nothing stopping one from being sent into the adult medicine exams.

The HEEADSSS Assessment

Undoubtedly, between now and publication, more Ds and Ss will be added into this acronym. This useful tool needs to be well known to the candidate. It covers the majority of issues faced by adolescents, with and without major health issues, all the way from Home to Safety.

Transition of Care

Moving from paediatrics to adult medicine is a massive change, for kids and their parents and carers (often the worst for parents!). Know about the transition process in your local area, and get along to transition clinics in action. This is all excellent long case fodder. It is a lot easier for you to talk about transition than the intricacies of Apert syndrome.

Problem: Teenagers still scare me. Help!

Solution: Channel your teenaged self.

You were a teenager once. Maybe you were a geek in the library trying to get into medical school. Maybe you hated school and were socially isolated. Maybe you were head girl, captain of the first netball team but had an eating disorder and a pregnancy scare at 16. Perhaps you were a goth-emo, rebelling against your neurologist parents. Maybe you quit the first XV, experimented wildly with drugs and alcohol and then got your life on track.

You don't have to share these experiences with anybody, but they will remind you of the pain and difficulties of adolescence and help you dig out some empathy when your 15-year-old patient ignores you under a curtain of hair and earphones. Channel whatever experiences you had as a teenager then… you guessed it… practise on real live ones. Get comfortable talking about sex, drugs, boys, girls, school, teachers, homosexuality, contraception, suicide, abuse and everything else. You, the candidate, must:

- be free from embarrasment
- have an approach that will remind you of the issues
- look like you've asked all these things before
- have actually talked to real live young people as patients and as practice cases
- be confident listening to embarrassing stuff
- have realistic strategies.

Summary

- Key goals for the paediatric long case: getting the patient onside, preventing boredom and gaining trust from the parent or carer.
- Get an approach to the common problems and challenges of childhood.
- Understand that different members of the family will have different concerns and priorities.
- It is important to identify realistic goals for every case: Educate, support, advocate, co-ordinate and optimise are your golden words.
- Developmental paediatrics terrifies many candidates as they may have limited experience. Think of a developmental assessment as a less structured, pragmatic assessment-something that an experienced general paediatrician would do every day.
- Have a flexible approach to getting a developmental history and examination. Make the most of spontaneous displays, and break out your official developmental examination to fill in obvious gaps or you will run out of time.
- Always think 'strengths and difficulties' for every part of the developmental case.
- Think of an adolescent long case as a gift – there is so much to talk about.
- Know your HEEADSSS assessment.
- Know the challenges of transitioning care and how you would solve them for your patient.
- Channel your inner teenager.
- Leave embarrassment at the door and be confident. Confidence can be learned with practice.

18

Secret Long Case Species

Everyone knows about the cardiovascular, transplant, developmental and adolescent long case categories. There are also secret species of long case which regularly throw candidates into disarray that you need to know about, and must be able to manage confidently and competently before Exam Day.

The secret species of long cases fall into four patterns:

- the chronic disease long case with multiple issues
- the single problem long case
- the diagnostic dilemma
- the disaster long case.

The Chronic Disease Long Case

These are not that bad to get, and they're what most candidates expect. Generally, the patient has enough issues to allow you to steer the discussion towards the topic that you understand the best.

For example, if you don't know much about amyloid but you do know about dialysis, then start your discussion by saying that 'dialysis is a very important issue for the patient' and spend as much time talking about this as possible. Often, the most important issue for the patient may not be related to their chronic problem but may be a treatment side effect, complication or something unrelated. Don't minimise or overlook these problems – make sure they are near the top of your problem list as the examiners will also want to focus on them.

How to Pass the RACP Written and Clinical Exams: The Insider's Guide,
Second Edition. Zoë Raos and Cheryl Johnson.
© 2017 John Wiley & Sons Ltd. Published 2017 by John Wiley & Sons Ltd.

The Single Problem Long Case

These are tough. You will have to know that one problem inside out and back to front because you are going to be answering questions about it for 10–20 minutes. Examples include a patient with IHD, asthma, anorexia nervosa or recent lymphoma. Shockers in recent times have included obscure single problems that even the patient can't pronounce. Generally speaking, most exam organisers will only list a single problem long case if there really is a lot to talk about. Even so, it pays to be prepared.

The trick with the single problem long case is to either come up with more problems from the social history or split the single problem into lots of little ones. For example, hepatitis B cirrhosis in a 54-year-old man. That is the only problem. There is no hypertension or anything else in the past medical history. The examination is unremarkable. The patient is employed and has a nice supportive family. Some candidates would freak out but if you think about it, there is actually loads to talk about:

- Staging of cirrhosis
- Assessing risk of decompensation
- Optimisation of antiviral medication
- Hepatocellular cancer surveillance
- Careful family screening
- Alcohol education
- Improve patient knowledge about universal precautions and being blood-safe in the home
- If you need to fill in time, you could talk about suitability for transplant (if the patient is well compensated this may be a bridge too far for some examiners)

Use up as much question time as possible by talking about the simple areas that don't require an indepth knowledge of the recent literature. Take the holistic route and talk about patient education, good follow-up arrangements and avoiding complications. Eventually they'll nail you with a question about cognition problems post-CABG surgery but hopefully that will be just as the bell is ringing.

The Diagnostic Dilemma Long Case

These aren't that common on Exam Day, but are very often encountered in your practice cases. They can come up on the day, though, so you need to be able to manage them. Think of shortness of breath as an example. Usually, the patient will have multiple reasons why they might be breathless and the examiners want to see you display a logical approach to investigating it. Make sure you have asked the patient the right questions to shorten your differential and have thought about what investigations you would want, so you can work out the cause of the symptom.

Even if you think you know the diagnosis, try and determine what the alternatives might be so you can discuss how you came to your conclusion.

Keep it simple. As per the short cases, list the simple, bedside investigations before the fancy radiology. Don't pull out the transthoracic echocardiogram looking for diastolic dysfunction before you mention the ECG looking for LVH and the FBC looking for anaemia.

If there really are 2–3 possible causes for the symptom, list the differentials in order from most likely to least likely. Discuss what supports or doesn't support each diagnosis. Discuss how there may be more than one cause. This approach can use up a large chunk of question time to excellent effect.

The Disaster Long Case

We can't tell you how to recover from a real-world disaster. One patient arrested in the middle of the long case, the candidate did CPR, hit the emergency bell, the resus crew arrived and the candidate passed (a red sticker was probably deployed, and the candidate kept her nerve for the rest of the long and short cases). A paediatric registrar had an adolescent long case patient who disclosed abuse for the first time in the middle of the history. The candidate handled it sensitively and effectively both with the patient and in the discussion, and passed with flying colours. Behind the scenes, exam organisers went into full Child Protection mode and deployed a cascade of support for the patient.

Disasters on an epic scale are rare. More commonly, medium-scale disasters derail candidates, and will do so for eternity. Be forewarned, and forearmed. Common disasters include:

- the patient with a disease you know nothing about
- the vague patient or the patient with unrecognised cognitive impairment
- the chatty patient
- the 'withholding information' patient
- the overly complex patient.

Disaster patients make your heart sink. Read on for advice, and take heart that the examiner probably had just as much trouble during their examination and will be eagerly waiting to see how you cope under the circumstances.

Dealing with Disaster: The Patient with a Disease You Know Nothing About

It could be amyloidosis, congenital anaemia, stem cell transplants … as soon as the patient says it, you panic. You start imagining how awful the discussion will be. Stop! Think! Keep your wits about you! This is one of the easier cases to pass:

1) **Present your findings logically**, even if you know nothing about the actual disease. Hopefully, the patient knows all about their disease and can guide you to what's important. Present chronologically, group admissions and procedures together and avoid parroting everything the patient told you.

> 'Patient has disease X which was diagnosed 10 years ago by…
> She takes … Medications…
> It has resulted in the following complications…
> She has had … Surgery for it…
> It is monitored by regular blood tests …'

2) **The examiners have probably never heard of it either** and have no idea of how to treat it. Your average examiner doesn't know their NNRTIs from their NRTIs so they are probably not going to grill you on it. They may ask you questions on general principles, so work out some general statements like 'I'd monitor for signs of infection in this immuno-suppressed patient'.
   If you are really stuck or don't know the answer, it is acceptable to say that you would consult your specialist colleagues for advice.

3) **The disease is probably not the reason why the patient is there.** Yes, they may have rhubarb-aemia but it's the patient's inability to work due to their lost driving licence that you are really meant to discover. Grill the patient for social issues, depression, functional limitations … anything that you can use in the discussion so that you can say 'Although they have Castleman's disease syndrome, the patient's major problems are depression and social isolation which I would like to discuss'.

Dealing with Disaster: The Vague Patient or Patient with Unrecognised Cognitive Impairment

Thankfully, these patients are rarely chosen by exam organisers, and if they turn up on the day, the examiners often (gently) reject them. But very occasionally, these patients can slip through the net, so be warned. You get an inkling that something is wrong when the patient can't remember what their disease is called. Further questioning just seems to make it worse, with the patient saying things like 'Yes, maybe it is called lipex or maybe losec or maybe Usee'.

1) Start with the **medication list** – this may help you work out what problems they might have so you can tailor your questions and examination.

2) **Do a MoCA and screen for depression and alcohol**. If the MoCA is significantly reduced, limit your time taking further history as it may be unreliable. Instead, focus on a social history to elicit any functional limitations that person may have followed by a super-thorough examination and then plan what you are going to say in the discussion.

3) Start your presentation by saying that patient had a MoCA of 15/30 and hence there may be **inaccuracies in the history** you are about to give. Don't say they were a poor historian or keep harping on about how difficult it was; say it once, say it clearly enough so they've got it, and then move on. No one likes a whingeing candidate!

4) Patient can't remember their pills? Great! This means that you can suck up half the discussion time by talking about their difficulties with **adherence to their medications**, their overly complicated medication administration regime and their poor understanding of their medical conditions. You'll be able to talk for ages about how you could improve compliance, and simplify medications into a blister pack.

5) If the MoCA is 30/30 yet your patient is incredibly sketchy on any details, **think of reasons why**. Perhaps cultural differences, lack of trust in the medical system, low education level or a language barrier are factors. Discuss this with the examiners, together with the importance of corroborative histories and old notes.

6) Be careful with the **language you use**. Describe the patient's deficiencies with sensitivity and tact and avoid derogatory statements.

Dealing with Disaster: The Chatty Patient

The patient who spends the whole time telling you about the war and you never get a word in edgewise to ask about their alcohol intake or home situation. Forty minutes are up and you are starting to panic that you aren't even going to finish the history, let alone examine them. Here are some tips:

1) When introducing yourself to the patient, make sure you tell them that **things are going to be rushed** and you are going to cut them off occasionally. Apologise in advance for doing this, and then try to be as firm as you can. (This is why you need to practise a few times; if you are a shy type you must learn to be assertive).
2) Use phrases like, 'Army, you say? Now tell me, do you smoke?' to help **move them along**.
3) Ask '**yes and no**' questions. The open-ended question has little or no place in this exam!

If all else fails, we have been known to **hold a hand up for 'stop'** or even 'time out'. Don't feel bad about this, it is your exam after all.

Dealing with Disaster: The 'Withholding Information' Patient

Some patients take delight in not giving you the information that you require. Whilst patients are 'coached' by examiners to answer questions openly but for reasons unclear they become evasive and vague. These are rare, as often such patients will not make it through the selection process but people are people, and people are strange.

1) Start with the **medication list** to get an idea of their problems.
2) Start with their main problem and work through subsequent problems as best you can. Be patient, and reassure the patient that they really can tell you everything.
3) In your discussion, be honest that you found the case to be a challenge, without whingeing (walk the line, the very fine line). Use this to any advantage you can, explaining how you would **establish more rapport** during subsequent consultations and get a corroborative history from the GP and family members. Then tackle other issues as best you can. Hopefully, the patient won't get asked back next year!

Dealing with Disaster: The Overly Complex Patient

They have 13 active medical problems, 24 different medications, have had 94 different types of surgery that you can't even spell … the history is spiralling out of control and every time you think you see the end, he hits you with 'and have I mentioned my liver transplant?'.

1) Start with the **medication list** to give you an idea of how much ground you have to cover.
2) Work out from the patient's medications what the **big diseases** are likely to be (transplant, diabetes, heart failure) so you don't get any surprises at the end.
3) Ask a few questions about each disease that seem relevant, then come back and **fill in the details at the end** once you've got an overview of important issues.
4) If the patient seems to have spent half their life in hospital having procedures, just ask about **the most recent ones or the most major ones**. Ask specifically about ones that might be important to you as a doctor (the answer to 'Have you had a nephrectomy?' is more important than the dates of their last four fistula blockages).
5) Keep asking questions while you are examining.
6) **Present succinctly** – you still have only 10 minutes to get through it all. Use wrap-up phrases like 'multiple presentations with febrile neutropenia and vascular access problems'.
7) There should be lots of scope to talk about polypharmacy, compliance with complicated drug regimes, difficulty with multiple doctor appointments, depression with constant admissions … make sure you mention these issues in your problem list.
8) Ask yourself, 'What is the point of this case? What is the number one issue facing this patient at this point in time?'. Always keep this in mind as there will be a specific reason why this case was selected.

Summary

- Secret species of long cases are not so scary when you're prepared for them. Know what they are, and how to get around them.
- Disaster long cases can actually be turned into a decent attempt if you keep your cool, think on your feet and have thought about an approach beforehand.
- Always ask yourself, 'What is the point of this case? Why was this particular person chosen?'.

19

Top Long Case Tips from Candidates and Examiners

Long Case Advice from Candidates

We asked as many registrars as possible to tell us their secrets to preparing and performing well in long cases. We received a range of handy hints that can help you:

- During your practice cases, ask for feedback on your style. Find out if you talk too fast or too quietly so you can practise changing this before the exam day.
- It's not about nailing. It's about not failing.
- Own the patient. Examiners love to hear statements like 'If Mr X was my patient, I would like to organise a …' or 'I would continue to review Mr X in my clinic and discuss sensitive issues further such as depression or impotence'. Don't try to palm the patient onto another subspecialist – you can consult with them but you don't have to refer every little thing.
- The open-ended question has no place in a long case! Keep your patients from rambling by asking yes/no or limited option questions.
- Don't feel like you need to mention every single thing that you found out about the patient, especially all the social stuff. Keep a few details up your sleeve so that you can pull them out during the discussion. This also allows your presentation to be more slick and 'to the point'. Just don't forget to mention them … if you don't talk about it, the examiners assume you didn't ask about it.

> 'Yes, it's interesting you mention weight loss strategies. We talked about this and I found out that she has recently looked into joining a gym.'

How to Pass the RACP Written and Clinical Exams: The Insider's Guide, Second Edition. Zoë Raos and Cheryl Johnson.
© 2017 John Wiley & Sons Ltd. Published 2017 by John Wiley & Sons Ltd.

- Don't slag off the patient. Even if they were the most annoying person in the world and you think they have ruined your chances of passing, try and remember that the patient didn't do it deliberately. At least try not to let the examiners realise that you feel like strangling the patient because this is very unprofessional.
- Be nice when you are talking about the patient. Helpful phrases include the following.

> 'The patient was reluctant to talk about that issue.'
> **Translation** – *I asked and they refused to answer.*
> 'I am concerned about the patient's understanding of his disease and the seriousness of his condition.'
> **Translation** – *the patient spent most of the interview reading a magazine.*
> 'The patient had difficulty remembering the names of his medications, raising the possibility of drug errors'.
> **Translation** – *The patient has no idea about his medical issues. At all.*
> 'The patient became agitated and tearful when talking about X. I felt it was inappropriate to continue this line of questioning until I had established better rapport with the patient.'
> **Translation** – *I totally put my foot in it and pissed off the patient.*

- Don't argue with the examiners (you are always wrong). Work out what is expected and achieve that. Yes, it's a bit too formal and a bit snooty and not like real life but that's how it is for exams and you do want to pass, after all.
- Obesity and cognitive problems frequently appear in a long case problem list so be prepared to talk about how you would approach them.
- The best long case ends up in a discussion rather than a Q and A session.
- If consultants tell you that you will pass and to stop doing practice cases then believe them! Don't fall for the line that you have to do 20 practice long cases. Everyone has their own threshold, but 7–12 seemed to be more than enough.
- It's quality not quantity when it comes to practice cases. Not every consultant is worth doing a practice long or short case with. Ask the people the year ahead who to avoid.

- Use the registrars who have just done their exams the previous year. They're probably better at doing cases than some of the consultants as they know the expected standard.
- Do at least one practice case with a past or current examiner.
- Don't think you have to quote studies to pass the long case. You're more likely to get tripped up in the details and look like an idiot. Only quote a study if you know it inside out. This is a test of your approach to a problem rather than whether you are able to recite an ARR from a recent study.
- Remember that common things appear commonly and often your long case victims will have at least one of these problems. (Common things aren't common in the short cases, though – in fact, that's entirely the opposite!)
- Go to an outpatient clinic for those specialties that don't have many inpatients, e.g. rheumatology or endocrinology. It's really useful if you've actually seen someone with scleroderma, nailfold infarcts, RA, etc. before Exam Day.
- Get a good rapport with the patient if you can. Some patients seem to think that they shouldn't just give the information and that the candidate should have to extract it from them. You have to have good rapport with them to get the good stuff! Try and finish within 40–45 minutes to allow yourself time to prepare and think.
- Think to yourself while you are writing your problem list:
  - 'What are they going to grill me on?'
  - 'What are the major/critical issues with this patient according to the patient and according to me as his physician?'
  - 'How can I make this patient take ownership and manage their own disease?'
  - Ask the patient 'Is there anything the examiners looked at or asked that I haven't?'
  - Ask the patient any questions that you forgot earlier.
- Remember to **cut the crap.** Don't waffle. They want all killer, no filler.
- During the long case, ask yourself the **key question** 'Why did they choose THIS case?' – answer that question and you will nail the case.
- Practise long cases with more senior registrars who are strong in the areas you struggle with. If you need to work on discussing management, practise cases with someone who makes it all sound beautiful. On the day, try to think how they would put things when preparing your discussion points!
- Consider the DeltaMed revision course. It is really good for long case discussions.

Long Case Advice from Examiners

We also asked examiners what they think helps in the long case. These people have watched hundreds of nervous registrars dig themselves into holes (then haul themselves out with varying degrees of success) so take their advice seriously!

- You need to present all your findings, including the problem list, in about 10–12 minutes and be ready to spend the rest of the time discussing the case. Avoid spending the whole presentation time laboriously listing the power in every muscle group. Practise your timing: history for 5–7 minutes, exam findings for 3–4 minutes max.
- Go through the medical problem list, medication history, social and family history, etc. without forgetting a single section!
- Practise with previous or current examiners.
- See lots of patients, and try to sound reflective and experienced on the day. They don't know that this is the first case of CREST you have ever seen.
- Give relevant negatives 'Importantly, there was no history of...'. Try not to give exhaustive lists of negatives, though.
- Always comment on the thyroid (e.g. 'not palpable'), skin, joints, back and gait (especially if relevant).
- Lying and standing blood pressure – do it.
- Practise with diabetics (diet, exercise, nurse reviews, eyes, podiatry, potency in males, waist measurements, blood glucose monitoring, timing of insulin/meds with relation to meals, driving, food in car, etc.). Mention secondary causes such as haemochromatosis and Cushing's.
- Get plenty of social history: the house set-up, stairs, home help, mobility, special societies, etc. Even if you don't say all this in your discussion, be prepared to pull out the details if asked.
- Think about the big picture rather than the details of the case. What is the main message about medicine that this patient personifies? Try to get this message across when you are presenting (though you don't need to say 'This is a classic textbook case of non-compliance' in your presentation!).
- Don't use abbreviations. It's confusing to listen to a long list of three-letter acronyms (BP/PND/DM/CAD). Don't assume that the examiner will instantly understand that MS stands for mitral

stenosis; they might spend half the case confused as to why you thought the patient had multiple sclerosis.

- Treat every new patient in clinic or ED as a long case. Don't read their notes before, start with their medication list and try to keep to time.
- Make sure you answer the question that is being asked. Don't manipulate the question into something else if you are not sure of the answer. It is better to say 'I don't know' rather than tangentially answer a question. Some examiners are 'like a dog with a bone' and will continually bring you back to the question until you have answered it.

20

Suggested Approach to a Māori Patient in the Long Case

Dr Matthew Wheeler, Advanced Trainee, Dunedin

Unfortunately, many health inequalities remain between Māori and non-Māori. This is your chance to show how you plan on addressing these inequalities one patient at a time. What follows are some brief suggestions. If you need more advice, we suggest contacting your hospital's Māori liaison support workers who might even offer you and your fellow candidates a tutorial. We were taught at medical school that a good grounding in Māori health will enable a doctor to generalise sensitivity to people of other cultures, and this is true. Think about the cultural needs of your Asian, African, Pacifican, Aboriginal and Torres Strait Island patients and include this in your long case preparation and discussion.

1) Ask them what ethnicity they are – let them self-identify. Assumption can end badly. On a recent ward round, a medical student assumed someone was Māori and the patient was actually Cambodian!
2) Ask the patient what iwi they are from, then ask them if it is from this area. If they don't know then that is also useful.
   'What is your iwi?' *Ngai Tahu.*
   'Sorry, I don't know about these things. Is that iwi from here?'
       No it's from the South Island.
3) Ask the patient if they are involved in their iwi in any way.
   'Are you involved in your iwi in any way?'
   'Do you have good whanau/family support?'
   'Is this your immediate or extended family?'

How to Pass the RACP Written and Clinical Exams: The Insider's Guide, Second Edition. Zoë Raos and Cheryl Johnson.

4) 'Did you get visits from the Māori liaison support workers when you are in hospital? Would you like to see them?'
5) Is your GP/GP practice a Māori health practice?

These questions allow you to gauge cultural connectedness. There is solid evidence that Māori who are connected are more supported and compliant with their healthcare than those who are not. This is important for your discussion. You can offer suggestions such as Māori support workers, a Māori health team, or a GP in a Māori health practice. All this helps with compliance and support.

6) 'Do you use any Māori medicine or healing? Would you like to have the opportunity for some?'
Examples include:
Mirimiri – massage
Romiromi – deep tissue massage and manipulation
Rongoa – herbal medicine. Could be important for drug interactions.

Putting it all Together

Mr R is a 56-year-old Māori man of Ngai Tahu descent who has diabetes that is poorly controlled. Along with his prescribed medication, he takes no traditional/Māori medicines or treatments. In terms of social history, Mr R currently lives outside his tribal areas and has no contact with his iwi. He has immediate whanau living locally but no extended support present. I note that although he identifies as Māori, he does not see the Māori support workers and has a non-Māori GP practice.

> **Paeds Point**
>
> 'Bonnie is a four-year-old girl of Tainui descent who is on the inpatient waiting list for a heart transplant. She usually lives with her immediate and extended whanau on family land in their own home. She is bilingual from attending kohanga reo, and mum's main educational concern for Bonnie is falling behind in her Te Reo because of all the trips to congenital heart clinic and indeterminate length of her current hospital stay. Bonnie and her whanau are well connected with her hapu and iwi. Bonnie's entire whanau are part of her transplant support team, particularly her Nan. This will be a real advantage for Bonnie in view of the precarious nature of her congenital heart disease and current place on the waiting list.'

In your plan, if you are feeling confident, incorporate the principles of the Whare Tapa Whā (four-sided house of wellness) into your discussion.

1) Tinana – physical health including traditional/Māori medicines
2) Hinengaro – mental health which can be addressed by talking with cultural workers
3) Wairua – spiritual health which can also be addressed by cultural workers or priest
4) **Whānau** – family health, including getting the family involved, educating them about the importance of their illness and compliance with treatment.

21

Long Case Examples

We have included four example long cases. They look long but take about 10 minutes to read out loud. It is impossible and unnecessary to write this level of detail for a live long case, but you can afterwards. We have included verbal signposts (in bold) but it is important to think what signposts you would use and try them out for yourself. It is economical to group diseases together.

These cases, presented as is, would get a solid 5 out of 7. As you will learn (the hard way), 6 and 7 grades come from the delivery. Have another look at the marking schedule. Being nimble with the examiners, showing the maturity of a junior consultant, confidence with eye contact and flexibility of thought are hard to put on paper. Don't put too much pressure on your performance when you start; remember, it's not about nailing, it's about not failing!

By reading this, you might understand better what we mean about terms like opening gambit and problem list. These examples are not the only way of presenting a long case, but give you a good foundation from which to develop your own style.

Long Case 1 – Multiple Medical Problem Management

Opening Gambit (Please note, you don't say 'opening gambit' out loud!)

Mrs P is a 66-year-old retired dressmaker with multiple medical problems including polycystic kidney disease, giant cell arteritis and polymyalgia rheumatica on long-term corticosteroid therapy, with

How to Pass the RACP Written and Clinical Exams: The Insider's Guide,
Second Edition. Zoë Raos and Cheryl Johnson.
© 2017 John Wiley & Sons Ltd. Published 2017 by John Wiley & Sons Ltd.

acromegaly and macular degeneration. Her life is severely restricted by loss of vision and she is a current heavy cigarette smoker.

Medical Problem List

Mrs P has a number of medical problems which I will discuss in turn.

At age 55, Mrs P was diagnosed with **macular degeneration**. Her first symptoms were zigzag lines in her central vision when driving. She was referred to an ophthalmologist who diagnosed her with macular degeneration. Her vision is now severely impaired and she stopped driving five years ago. She is able to differentiate colours and shape outlines but has difficulty with reading and identifying people or items. She is treated with monthly bevacizumab injections, and is seen regularly in the ophthalmology clinic.

Mrs P was diagnosed with **acromegaly** four years ago. It was her sister who prompted her to see her GP as she noticed a change in appearance. Mrs P herself had noticed an increase in the size of her hands, feet and tongue and she had to have her rings cut off due to finger swelling. Her GP referred her to an endocrinologist who arranged an MRI brain which revealed a pituitary mass. She underwent transsphenoidal resection of the pituitary tumour which was completed without complication. She is followed up with two-yearly MRI brain scans and these have not demonstrated any recurrence. Mrs P has had intermittent frontal headaches since the surgery. She does not have a visual field defect. She has not had any problems with other aspects of the pituitary axis, in particular she has no thyroid or cortisol dysfunction.

Following the pituitary surgery, Mrs P was found to have an abdominal mass. USS revealed **polycystic kidneys and liver**. She reports normal renal and liver function, and she is monitored regularly with blood and urine tests. She is not troubled by abdominal pain. She has not been investigated for cerebral aneurysms, nor has she been diagnosed with mitral valve prolapse, but her general practitioner recently noticed a heart murmur and she has been referred for an echocardiogram. Her family have not been affected to her knowledge.

Mrs P was diagnosed with both **giant cell arteritis** and polymyalgia rheumatica two years ago. Her presenting symptoms were hip and shoulder girdle pain, as well as headaches and bitemporal tenderness, but she did not have jaw claudication. She had no new associated visual symptoms. Her ESR was raised and she was started on high-dose corticosteroid therapy which has since been tapered and she is currently on 4 mg. She does experience occasional pain symptoms in her shoulder and hip girdles and she is not sure of her current ESR. In terms of **corticosteroid-related side effects**, Mrs P was diagnosed with osteoporosis on a screening bone mineral density scan last year. She has never had a fracture, and is not prone to falling. She is treated with vitamin D and a bisphosphonate. Her skin has thinned on treatment and she bruises easily. Her weight has remained relatively stable but she has developed abdominal striae.

Mrs P has an **essential tremor** affecting her head and limbs that has been present since childhood and worsened during puberty. She has been on propranolol for many years for this after review by a neurologist. There is no familial history of essential tremor and her tremor does improve if she drinks alcohol.

Medications (Grouped by Indication and Importance)

Mrs P's **current medications** are:

- prednisone 4 mg daily
- omeprazole 20 mg daily
- citalopram 20 mg daily
- lorazepam 0.5 mg nocte
- propranolol 40 mg twice daily
- folic acid 5 mg daily
- iron tablets 325 mg daily
- calciferol 1.25 mg monthly
- zoledronate infusions two yearly
- bevacizumab injection.

Mrs P does not use blister packs and reports good compliance. She has no known drug allergies or intolerances. She has a yearly influenza vaccination but has not had the pneumococcal vaccination.

Social History

In terms of **social history**, Mrs P lives in Beachlands with her husband of 46 years. He is unwell with an invasive skin cancer and is currently awaiting surgery. They own their own home. Five years ago, Mr P's business collapsed and they lost a significant amount of money so had to refinance their home. This has been incredibly stressful for the family.

Mrs P has two children who live in Auckland and three grandchildren. She worked as a dress maker, and quit around five years ago due to her deteriorating vision. She was also a keen keyboard player which she gave up as she was no longer able to read music. Mrs P still enjoys crocheting. Although she is unable to drive, she rides a three-wheeled bicycle to the shops which gives her independence.

Mrs P is a current heavy smoker with a 40 pack/year history. She has no diagnosis of chronic airways disease and has never been admitted to hospital with a chest infection.

She is up to date with her screening mammograms and cervical smears which have been normal.

Mrs P is taking citalopram and benzodiazepine for **depression** and anxiety, diagnosed around the time of the family business collapsing and the stress of the financial hardship. However, with time passing she is feeling better about this and is interested in coming off these medications. She denies vegetative symptoms of depression and has no suicidal thoughts. She reports her appetite and sleep patterns are normal.

She has a good relationship with her general practitioner who she visits regularly.

Family History

In terms of **family history**, Mrs P is the fourth oldest of 11 children. Surprisingly, there is no significant family history, including polycystic kidney disease or essential tremor.

Examination

On **examination**, Mrs P is a woman who looks older than her 66 years. She did not have cushingoid facies. She appeared comfortable at rest. Her peripheries were warm and well perfused with palmar erythema and wasting of the intrinsic muscles of the hands and the thenar and hypothenar eminences. Her skin appeared thin and she had multiple bruises over the hands and forearms.

Respiration rate was 16 breaths per minute, radial pulse rate was 70 beats per minute and clinically in sinus rhythm. Blood pressure was 158/70 lying and 160/75 standing.

Visual acuity was 6/18 in the left eye, and counting fingers on the right. Visual fields were difficult to interpret but I did not find a clear visual field defect. Undilated fundoscopy was attempted but I did not get adequate views.

Carotid pulse was of normal character and the jugular venous pressure was measured at 1 cm. Heart sounds were dual with an ejection systolic murmur loudest at the apex which radiated to the axilla and was enhanced with expiration but not with Valsalva manoeuvre. There was no click audible. The murmur was also audible at the base of the heart but did not radiate to the carotids. Her chest was clear with no wheeze or crackles.

The abdomen was asymmetrical in appearance and there was a large mass on the right consistent with an enlarged liver measured at 17 cm. I could not palpate the kidneys bilaterally. There was no ascites.

Neurological examination was unremarkable; notably, there was no proximal muscle weakness.

Summary Statement

In summary, Mrs P is a 66-year-old woman with the management problems of visual impairment secondary to macular degeneration, giant cell arteritis and polymyalgia rheumatica on long-term corticosteroid therapy with the complication of osteoporosis and untreated hypertension, along with the diagnostic problems of polycystic kidney disease and new ejection systolic murmur, and the social problem of heavy smoking.

Problem List

There are **eight problems** that I would like to discuss further.

1) Visual loss and the significant impact on Mrs P's daily activities and life
2) Essential tremor which according to Mrs P is her biggest problem
3) Polycystic kidney disease and potential for renal failure
4) Continued heavy smoking and the associated health implications
5) Diagnosis of the new ejection systolic murmur
6) Hypertension which is inadequately treated
7) Long-term steroid use and osteoporosis
8) Management of her mood issues

Problem	Differential diagnosis	Investigations	Management
Visual loss most likely secondary to macular degeneration	Optic chiasm compression or trauma from pituitary microadenoma +/− surgery Cataracts due to intercurrent corticosteroid use	Review old notes regarding diagnosis of pituitary tumour and macular degeneration, including operative notes and ophthalmology assessment Review brain MRI scans	Bevacizumab injections Referral to Foundation for the Blind Half-price taxi chits Personal care support/ domiciliary support may be needed in future Compliance stated as good, but need to discuss blister packs
Essential tremor	Parkinsonism/ early symptoms Parkinson's disease Medication related Exacerbated by low mood	Routine bloods including thyroid function	Treat with propranolol titrated to symptoms Acknowledge this as a difficult problem, reassurance Ongoing observation and input from MDT
Polycystic kidney disease and potential for renal failure	Simple renal cysts	Bloods including renal function with creatinine and eGFR and liver function including synthetic function Urinary albumin: creatinine ratio Review previous abdominal imaging and MRI brain imaging in particular MRA	Manage hypertension to preserve renal function with ACE inhibitor Ongoing observation with regular measurement of renal and liver function Genetic testing, consider family screening

Problem	Differential diagnosis	Investigations	Management
Current smoker with 40 pack/year history	At risk of smoking-related airways disease and cardiovascular disease as well as malignancy	Spirometry +/− pulmonary function tests Chest X-ray to exclude malignancy or signs of chronic airways disease Assess cardiovascular risk with lipid profile and HbA1c along with an ECG More functional tests including an ETT or echo may be warranted	Discuss benefits of quitting smoking and provide educational material Currently in the precontemplative phase Once ready, phone counselling through QuitLine would be helpful plus medical therapy with NRT or varenicline if NRT fails although reluctant while on SSRI
Ejection systolic murmur clinically most consistent with mitral regurgitation	MVP given PCKD AS/aortic sclerosis TR although no peripheral signs to support this	ECG looking for evidence of LV hypertrophy Chest X-ray looking for cardiomegaly or evidence of cardiac failure Echocardiogram to assess murmur	Examiners will give results, so candidate thinks on feet according to these
Hypertension	Essential hypertension Related to PCKD Complication of corticosteroid therapy Secondary HTN less likely	Assessment of cardiovascular risk as previously mentioned Consider secondary HTN work-up	Exercise and weight loss Stopping smoking ACE inhibition in the first instance

(Continued)

(Continued)

Problem	Differential diagnosis	Investigations	Management
Osteoporosis		Assess creatinine clearance and suitability for IV bisphosphonate therapy Review BMD scan Calculate FRAX score to determine 10-year fracture risk and determine need for bisphosphonate therapy	IV bisphosphonate therapy if appropriate based on creatinine clearance and FRAX score Continue vit D Weight-bearing exercise through MDT Aim for lowest prednisone dose to control GCA/PMR symptoms
Mood issues and management	Stressors include financial hardship, ill husband, continued loss of vision and impact on life Effect of corticosteroids on mood	States mood stable, need ongoing appointments, corroborative history from GP/family and rapport Consider a Depression Score	Social work/counselling Financial aid if appropriate +/- Citizen's Advice Bureau for budgeting advice Additional home support may be needed during Mr P's surgery Discuss discontinuation of therapy as identified by patient Attempt to taper benzodiazepine first due to problems with long-term use

Long Case 2 – Complicated Diabetes Case

Opening Gambit

Thank you for asking me to see Mr S, a 62-year-old retired banker who is currently an inpatient for treatment of an infected left diabetic foot ulcer. This is on a background of long-standing type 2 diabetes mellitus with multiple micro- and macrovascular complications, and the social problem of inability to work secondary to his foot ulcer.

Medical Problem List

Mr S was diagnosed with **type 2 diabetes** 16 years ago after presenting to his general practitioner with fatigue. He had also several urinary tract infections and noted cuts that were slow to heal in the two years leading up to this. Random glucose taken at the time was 23. He was referred to an endocrinologist who started low-dose metformin and gliclazide; the doses of these have been increased since then, but he has never been on insulin and he is not keen on injections.

He reports good **blood sugar control**, with most recent HbA1c of 52. He does not do capillary glucose testing and denies **hypoglycaemic events** on his current treatment regimen.

The main **complication** of his long-standing diabetes is diabetic foot ulcers. He first had an ulcer on the plantar aspect of the left forefoot 14 years ago. This started as a blister and was treated with intravenous antibiotics in hospital, had district nurse dressing for 12 months and did not require surgery. He had no further problems until one month ago when he developed blisters on the balls of both feet. Mr S attributes this to starting a new job where he is on his feet for eight hours three days per week. The blisters have now broken down to ulcers and he was recently treated with seven days of flucloxacillin by his GP. The left ulcer is painful but has improved with starting nortriptyline. On a visit to the podiatry clinic yesterday, the left ulcer was noted to still be infected and the wound could be probed to the bone so he was admitted to hospital. He has been started on IV clindamycin and last night had debridement surgery.

Other **microvascular complications** include diabetic retinopathy found shortly after he was diagnosed with diabetes, along with glaucoma. He had retinal laser treatment within the first year of diagnosis but none since. He has yearly retinal screening. He states his vision is unchanged.

Mr S is not aware of having nephropathy and has regular blood tests with creatinine monitored by his GP. His last urine albumin:creatinine ratio was normal two weeks ago. He denies symptoms of autonomic neuropathy, including postural dizziness, diarrhoea or erectile dysfunction.

Macrovascular complications include cerebrovascular disease. Mr S had two transient ischaemic attacks that occurred within three days of each other seven years ago. Symptoms included left-sided facial weakness and expressive dysphasia for a few minutes. He was investigated with electrocardiogram, CT head, carotid Doppler and echocardiogram; he understands these were normal. Aspirin and dipyridamole were started.

He is not aware of a diagnosis of ischaemic heart disease. He does not experience angina or symptoms of heart failure. Cardiac risk factors in addition to diabetes include hypertension and past smoking history.

More recently, Mr S's GP has told him he is **anaemic** with haemoglobin of 100, down from 150 six months ago. He denies melaena or fresh rectal bleeding. He has been fatigued for the last month but has not been breathless on exertion or experienced any chest pain. He is not a vegetarian and eats meat regularly. He had not noticed any change in bowel habit. He has lost 12 kg in the six months since starting his job, which he attributes to the long hours walking. He is concerned about his weight loss.

Medications

In terms of his **current medications**, he is taking:

- gliclazide 80 mg bd
- metformin 850 mg bd
- aspirin 100 mg daily
- dipyridamole 150 mg twice daily
- simvastatin 40 mg daily
- cilazapril 2.5 mg daily
- nortriptyline 20 mg nocte
- paracetamol regularly
- OxyNorm prn
- clindamycin 600 mg IV four times daily to treat wound infection
- bimatoprost eye drops.

He has no known drug **allergies** and reports good **compliance** with medications which are blister packed. He does not receive an annual influenza vaccination.

Social History

In terms of **social history**, Mr S lives with his wife and adult daughter in their own home in Whangaparaoa. He has a two-storey house with 15 stairs. They moved from Wellington one year ago after his wife was made redundant and found a new job in Auckland. They have two other daughters aged 25 and 27 who live in Auckland also. Their eldest daughter suffers from mental illness, including depression and a personality disorder; she is on a sickness benefit and lives with Mr S and his wife where she will likely remain as she requires their full-time support. This is very difficult for the family at times.

Mr S worked for ANZ Bank for 40 years and retired five years ago. Since moving to Auckland, he has taken up a part-time job working as a security guard at Woolworths. It is unlikely that he will be able to return to work when discharged from hospital. Mr S is not particularly concerned about the financial implications of losing his job but will miss the social interaction of going to work as well as the satisfaction of contributing to the household.

He drives and is independent with his daily activities, and is an active member of the local bridge club. He has a 40 pack/year smoking history and quit when diagnosed with diabetes after some 'stern words' from his endocrinologist. He drinks two units of alcohol once a week for the last two months, but over the years he has been a heavy drinker, drinking 30–40 units per week while working for ANZ.

He has a good relationship with his GP. He denies any depressive symptoms.

In terms of **family history**, Mr S's wife and daughter have both been diagnosed with type 2 diabetes this year and are managed with medications. Neither of his parents had diabetes, but his paternal grandfather did and used insulin from a young age. There is no significant family history of cardiovascular disease.

On **examination**, Mr S is of average build and appeared comfortable at rest. His left leg was elevated on pillows and a vacuum dressing was in place. He was warm and well perfused peripherally. His pulse rate was 76 beats per minute and he was clinically in sinus rhythm. His blood pressure was 135/85 with no postural drop. His JVP was measured at 1 cm and his carotid pulse was of normal character. His heart sounds were dual with no added sounds. His respiratory examination was unremarkable, as was his abdominal examination except for increased abdominal girth.

On examination of his peripheral vascular system, his feet were warm but with sluggish capillary refill. His posterior tibial and dorsalis pedis pulses were present but diminished. His nails were atrophic and thickened. The skin over his lower legs had lost its hair and was shiny. He had no peripheral oedema or varicose veins. He had a vacuum dressing over the plantar aspect of his left foot and his ulcer was not reviewed today.

On examination of his peripheral nerves, his knee jerks were normal but his ankle jerks were diminished in comparison. He had evidence of a stocking neuropathy with loss of vibration sensation to his knees bilaterally and light touch and pinprick sensation was diminished to the mid-shin bilaterally. His proprioception was normal.

On undilated fundoscopic examination, I was unable to appreciate any cataracts but had limited views of his fundi.

Summary Statement

In summary, Mr S is a 62-year-old part-time security guard and avid bridge player with the management problem of a left infected diabetic foot ulcer, on the background of long-standing type 2 diabetes with multiple micro- and macrovascular complications.

Problem List

Regarding Mr S's ongoing management, I have identified **five main problems**.

1) Immediate treatment and long-term management of the infected diabetic foot ulcer and peripheral neuropathy
2) Long-standing type 2 diabetes with complications including retinopathy and possible undiagnosed nephropathy
3) Diagnosis and management of his newly identified anaemia and weight loss
4) Poor engagement with health services since arriving in Auckland with subsequent deterioration in health and diabetic complications
5) Inability to work due to health conditions and the financial and social implications of this

Problem	Differential diagnosis	Investigations	Management
Diabetic foot ulcer	Arterial vs venous vs neuropathic ulcer	Routine blood tests including full blood count and inflammatory markers Wound swab X-ray right foot to assess for osteomyelitis MRI right foot to determine extent of infection MRA legs to determine extent of vascular disease	Debridement of ulcer and determine extent of infection. Liaise with specialist surgeon daily IV antibiotics Vacuum dressing to aid healing, specialist wound nurse care, at risk of pressure areas Elevation Enoxaparin and VTE prophylaxis measures Revascularisation as appropriate Podiatry input and orthotics review for footwear Education regarding peripheral neuropathy and foot care if needed
Type 2 diabetes		Routine blood tests including HbA1c and renal function Urinary microalbumin: creatinine ratio Review results of retinal screening Review diagnosis with anti-GAD and IA2 antibodies Assess cardiovascular risk with fasting lipids, ECG and chest X-ray	Uptitrate ACE inhibitor to control hypertension and proteinuria Ongoing monitoring of microvascular complications Regular HbA1c measurement May need to introduce insulin in future, offer education and diabetes nurse specialist input Optimise cardiovascular risk with dietary modification, alcohol reduction, exercise and optimisation of statin

(Continued)

(Continued)

Problem	Differential diagnosis	Investigations	Management
Newly identified anaemia	Iron or B12/folate deficiency Anaemia of chronic disease/ inflammation Broad differential for anaemia	Review FBC, in particular haemoglobin and MCV/blood film Iron studies, vitamin B12/folate, thyroid and liver function, inflammatory markers, coeliac antibodies, serum protein electrophoresis, immunoglobulins	If iron deficient, will need further investigation to exclude GI blood loss with colonoscopy/ gastroscopy Replace iron/B12/folate if appropriate (this is part of discussion where the candidate thinks on feet depending on investigation results)
Poor engagement with health services			Optimise rapport with patient, make repeat appointment as his general physician Ensure regular retinal screening and podiatry input booked Engage GP/practice nurse and set up regular review Engage diabetes nurse specialist and dietician for follow-up and support Regular clinic review Patient education regarding disease if needed
Inability to work			Review with occupational therapist – is it realistic for him to return to his role? Manage underlying problem and orthotic input for adequate footwear Social work input Financial assistance if needed Discussion with employer regarding changed duties, return to work programme Consider alternative employment or volunteer work to maintain social engagement

Long Case 3 – Diagnostic Long Case

Opening Gambit

Mrs H is a 73-year-old retirement village resident and retired motel owner who has been admitted to hospital with a syncopal episode thought secondary to dehydration from vomiting and diarrhoea. Mrs H has a background of long-standing rheumatoid arthritis and polymyalgia rheumatica, chronic pain issues and ischaemic heart disease. She has concerns about how her medical problems will impact on her independence.

Medical Problem List

Mrs H has been troubled with alternating **constipation and diarrhoea** following recent hip joint replacement surgery. She presented to hospital with a **syncopal episode** following multiple episodes of vomiting and diarrhoea. Mrs H woke the previous morning with nausea followed by abrupt-onset vomiting. She subsequently developed profuse diarrhoea with watery bowel motions without blood or mucus. Her bowels opened six times in the preceding 24 hours, including two episodes overnight. Whilst walking to the toilet to move her bowels, Mrs H felt lightheaded and dizzy and collapsed to the ground. She had no other preceding symptoms. She had a brief loss of consciousness before waking on the floor but was aware of her surroundings. Nursing staff in the retirement village reported no significant confusion following the syncopal episode with no evidence of seizure activity, including incontinence or tongue biting. The ambulance was called and on their arrival, she had improved with normal observations. She has never had a syncopal episode in the past. Investigations completed in hospital have revealed a normal ECG with no new changes, normal abdominal X-ray and a CT abdomen and stool samples are pending.

This recent episode is on the background of **alternating constipation and diarrhoea** for the last two months following her right total hip joint replacement. Since her surgery, Mrs H has had episodes of watery profuse diarrhoea followed by several days of not passing any bowel motions and then further episodes of diarrhoea. There has been no blood or mucus seen in the bowel motion. Mrs H has **lost weight** following her operation but is unable to quantify exactly how much. Her appetite was initially poor postoperatively but has gradually improved over the last six weeks.

Mrs H's other main concern is **chronic back and right hip pain** on a background of **rheumatoid arthritis and polymyalgia rheumatica**. Her pain started eight years ago and has worsened over that time. She was initially managed with simple analgesia, including paracetamol and non-steroidal anti-inflammatory medications. She was subsequently seen by an orthopaedic surgeon and was diagnosed with **nerve root entrapment** coupled with severe right hip **osteoarthritis**. She underwent an MRI scan of her lumbar spine which confirmed multilevel nerve root involvement predominantly on the right side. She was started on gabapentin and oxycodone but had significant side effects with treatment, including opioid-induced constipation and gabapentin-related drowsiness. As a result, her quality of life has been severely impacted due to pain and adverse drug-related effects.

Mrs H underwent a **right hip joint replacement** in March 2014 due to worsening pain. Her surgery was complicated by a large right hip haematoma which was managed conservatively with red blood cell transfusion. Postoperatively, she has had significant **right hip pain** which has been managed with oxycodone. She is currently able to mobilise with the aid of a frame when walking outside and a stick or unaided inside.

Mrs H was diagnosed with **rheumatoid arthritis and polymyalgia rheumatica** 10 years ago by a private rheumatologist. She **initially presented** with bilateral hand polyarthritis along with bilateral shoulder and hip girdle pain. She was **first commenced** on hydroxychloroquine and prednisone. She gradually tapered the prednisone dose and is currently on 5 mg. She has not been trialled on methotrexate.

After initially being managed in the private sector, four years ago Mrs H was discharged to the care of her general practitioner. Since then, she has been troubled by occasional joint 'flares' particularly affecting her hands and feet which are managed with an increase in her steroid dose. She has morning stiffness of up to 30 minutes. She does not have a clear action plan in the event that she develops worsening joint symptoms.

In terms of **steroid complications**, Mrs H has two-yearly zoledronate infusions and her most recent bone mineral density scan six months ago showed an increase in her T-score. She has also gained weight on prednisone and has problems of skin fragility and easy bruising. Her family history is notable for rheumatoid arthritis.

In terms of **other active problems**, Mrs H was admitted to hospital with a late presentation myocardial infarct in 1985 at the age of 45 years. She was managed medically but continued to have exertional angina for many years. She subsequently underwent a three-vessel coronary artery bypass graft at the age of 59 years for unstable angina. Currently, her symptoms are well managed and she uses her nitrolingual spray 2–3 times a year. Her exercise tolerance is limited by back and right hip pain rather than angina or shortness of breath. As part of her anaesthetic assessment for the right total hip joint replacement, Mrs H had a normal transthoracic echocardiogram and dobutamine stress echocardiogram.

In terms of **other medical problems**, Mrs H was diagnosed with depression two years ago and was initiated on paroxetine. She has also had two basal cell carcinomas resected from her lower legs due to historical sun exposure.

Medications

In terms of her **current medications**, Mrs H is on:

- gabapentin 200 mg tds
- OxyContin 10 mg bd with OxyNorm 5 mg as needed for break-through pain
- paracetamol 1 g four times daily
- paroxetine 20 mg daily
- aspirin 100 mg daily
- GTN spray as needed for angina
- hydrocortisone 50 mg IV q4h due to vomiting but is usually on prednisone 5 mg
- hydroxychloroquine 200 mg daily
- cholecalciferol 1.25 mg monthly
- zoledronate infusion two yearly
- diarrhoea being managed acutely with IV cefuroxime and metronidazole and she is on enoxaparin as DVT prophylaxis

She has no known drug **allergies** and reports good **compliance** with medications which are blister packed. She had her influenza vaccination this year but has not had a pneumococcal vaccination. She takes fish oil capsules and glucosamine with chondroitin as over-the-counter medications.

Social History

In terms of **social history**, Mrs H lives in a villa in a retirement village with her husband. Her husband had a stroke last year but does not require any assistance from Mrs H for his personal care. Prior to their retirement eight years ago, they owned and managed a motel. They have two children, both of whom live in Auckland and provide good social support. Despite her medical conditions, Mrs H maintains a busy social life and enjoys playing petanque and attending tai chi for physical exercise. Mrs H still drives. She is an ex-smoker, having stopped 40 years ago, but has a 20 pack/year history. She does not drink alcohol. She remained independent with her finances and receives a pension. Mrs H has home care provided by the Salvation Army three times a week for housework and supervision with showering. She has a good relationship with her general practitioner. Her insight into her medical problems is excellent but she has not yet completed an advance care plan. Her daughter is her Enduring Power of Attorney for both health/welfare and property which is not currently activated.

Family History

Mrs H's **family history** is notable for rheumatoid arthritis affecting her mother and aunt. Her mother died at the age of 83 years. Her father died of what was thought to be a myocardial infarct in his mid-50s.

Examination

On **examination,** Mrs H is well groomed and in no apparent distress. She has evidence of **steroid-related side effects** including truncal obesity and thin skin with multiple bruises on her forearms. On examination of her hands, she has ulnar deviation bilaterally with symmetrical polyarticular deformities affecting the metacarpophalangeal and proximal interphalangeal joints. There were no nail changes. She has no evidence of active synovitis. She is significantly **functionally limited** and is unable to undo buttons or hold a key.

On examination of her **eyes**, she has cataracts bilaterally but no fundoscopic abnormalities. She has a central scotoma on visual field testing. She has top and bottom dentures. On examination of her **cardiorespiratory** system, her pulse rate was 75 beats per minute and regular. Her blood pressure was 100/60 with no postural drop. On examination of her JVP, she has prominent venous pulsations but her jugular venous pressure was 1 cm. She has no carotid bruit. On examination of her anterior chest, she has a midline sternotomy scar. Her heart sounds were dual with no added sounds. Her chest was clear to auscultation. She has a left leg saphenous vein harvest scar.

On examination of her **abdomen**, she has a cholecystectomy scar. She has mild generalised abdominal tenderness with normal bowel sounds. I did not complete a rectal examination today but would wish to complete this as part of my examination. On examination of her right hip, her wound has healed well but there is significant soft tissue swelling with a degree of residual palpable haematoma.

Her **neurological examination** was unremarkable and in particular there was no proximal myopathy.

Summary Statement

In **summary**, Mrs H is a 73-year-old retirement village resident who, despite her significant medical problems, remains staunchly independent. She presents with the **diagnostic problems** of syncope and alternating diarrhoea and constipation. This is on a background of rheumatological disease with pain symptoms requiring long-term corticosteroids with significant treatment-related side effects. Her main **social concern** is her wish to remain independent but she recognises the impact that her significant medical problems pose, both currently and in the future.

Problem List

There are **seven problems** that I would like to discuss.

1) Syncope with brief loss of consciousness
2) Change in bowel habit following hip joint replacement surgery
3) Complications following her recent hip joint replacement surgery
4) Chronic back and hip pain and effect on quality of life
5) Steroid-related side effects
6) Treatment-related side effects and monitoring
7) Advance care planning

Problem	Differential diagnosis	Investigations	Management
Syncope with brief loss of consciousness	Dehydration secondary to GI losses Postural hypotension exacerbated by inability to absorb corticosteroids Cardiac arrhythmia or myocardial infarct	Routine blood tests including full blood count, renal function and inflammatory markers Lying/standing blood pressure Electrocardiogram Cardiac monitoring Medication review	Rehydration therapy Treat underlying diarrhoea illness Issues around driving Ongoing monitoring for further syncopal episodes (discussion will depend on investigation results given to the candidate)
Change in bowel habit	Mixed diarrhoea/ constipation Faecal overflow with underlying constipation secondary to opioids Gastroenteritis Bowel malignancy Inflammatory bowel disease or microscopic colitis *Clostridium difficile* infection	Routine blood tests including renal function and inflammatory markers Stool sample for microscopy, culture and *Clostridium difficile* infection Abdominal X-ray to exclude faecal loading/impaction Further investigations may include faecal calprotectin, steatocrit, pancreatic elastase, coeliac antibodies Colonoscopy +/− biopsy CT colonography less useful for investigation of diarrhoea	Rehydration therapy Rationalise antibiotics – treat infection only if demonstrated on stool specimens Cefuroxime and metronidazole broad spectrum and put patient at risk of *C.difficile* Medication review, uptitrate gabapentin if possible, rationalise opioids Oral and rectal laxatives to treat impaction if present Treat any other conditions found, including inflammatory bowel disease

Problem	Differential diagnosis	Investigations	Management
Complications following recent hip surgery	Development of haematoma and subsequent pain	Full blood count and anticoagulation status monitoring Iron studies Review results of hip imaging either CT/MRI Review operation notes and perioperative care	Transfusion to keep haemoglobin >90 g/dL If iron deficiency then will need iron replacement therapy Discuss plan with orthopaedic surgeon Analgesia Mobilisation Physiotherapy and use of appropriate walking aid Occupational therapy review regarding ability to manage at home
Chronic back and hip pain and effect on quality of life	Complex and multifactorial Right hip osteoarthritis Spinal nerve root compression or spinal stenosis Musculoskeletal Insufficiency fracture Bony metastatic disease Multiple myeloma	Routine blood tests including myeloma screen and inflammatory markers Review results relating to diagnosis of RA/PMR including anti-CCP antibodies, rheumatoid factor and ANA, along with inflammatory markers and bilateral hand X-rays Lumbar spine and hip X-rays MRI lumbar spine +/− hip and sacrum Review results of recent bone mineral density scan	Manage patient expectations: emphasise this is a **management issue** and a quick fix is unlikely Analgesia review, uptitrate gabapentin, reduce opioids Exercise programme and strength/balance training, and encourage ongoing petanque and tai chi Physiotherapy review and provision of an appropriate walking aid, hydrotherapy Review need for increased personal care assistance Monitor for worsening depressive symptoms Consider referral to Regional Pain Service for full package of MDT care

(Continued)

(Continued)

Problem	Differential diagnosis	Investigations	Management
Steroid-related side effects	Osteoporosis Thin skin Easy bruising Immuno-suppression Diabetes monitoring	Review bloods including HbA1c Review results of recent bone mineral density scan	Fall prevention strategies including physiotherapy, provision of an appropriate walking aid plus occupational therapy home assessment Hip protectors Zoledronate infusion if appropriate Exercise and wellness programme Dietary and weight control advice Continue to actively taper prednisone to lowest possible dose Review action plan for illness Influenza/pneumococcal vaccination
Treatment-related side effects and monitoring	Hydroxy-chloroquine Gabapentin Oxycodone	Review results of retinal screening Regular vision assessment	Rationalise and review medications regularly Consider effects of medication on driving ability and mobility
Advance care planning/care planning for the future	Discuss her wishes for care at end of life/in the event of deterioration		Compassionate discussion of long-term prognosis and planning for deteriorating health or changes in the future May need an increased level of care in the future Regular review

Long Case 4 – Adolescent Single Problem Long Case with Transition of Care

Opening Gambit

Thomas is a 16-year-old young man with steroid-dependent Crohn's disease requiring surgery at the age of 12, with a rocky course since then. He also has issues including failure to thrive with small stature, anaemia, acne and social difficulties, including being bullied and falling behind his classmates at school. Tom's main concern is being sick all the time and teasing, and his mother's main concern is his educational future and the long-term effects of his immune suppression therapy.

Medical Problem List

Tom's first medical problem is **steroid-dependent Crohn's disease** with ongoing symptoms suggesting poor control. This presented after a year of undiagnosed abdominal pain and diarrhoea, during which time his family sought treatment with complementary medicine. Tom presented acutely on his 13th birthday to the Royal Children's Hospital with severe pain from a bowel obstruction, and subsequently had an open ileocaecal resection. He is unsure how much bowel was removed. Unfortunately, he had a stormy postoperative course, including wound dehiscence and collections, and had a defunctioning ileostomy for 12 months which was then reversed. Tom and his family struggled to cope with the stoma; mum states 'he is never having surgery again'. He went to school one day and the bag burst, causing significant embarrassment for Tom.

His **Crohn's disease is managed** with a combination of mesalazine, azathioprine and prednisone (current dose 15 mg; he has been taking this fairly continuously for 24 months). He also sees a number of alternative health practitioners. He is unable to recall when he last had a colonoscopy but he had an MRI scan of the abdomen six months ago.

Tom describes pain many times per day, worse after eating high-fibre foods and vegetables. He is currently on a raw food diet on the advice of a naturopath which he thinks makes him feel worse and he prefers plain food. The family have seen a hospital dietician, but are going with the naturopath's advice currently.

The next problem is **low mood and a fairly conflicted relationship with his specialists**. When I spoke with Tom by himself for part of the history, he expressed how he is 'sick of being sick', 'sick of mum and dad fighting with the doctors with me like piggy in the middle' with different appointments with different professionals all giving him different advice. Tom likes his naturopath (John) and one of the gastroenterology registrars at the hospital. He thought about ending his life especially when he had the stoma, but denies overt depression and just wants to be like his friends. He is **ambivalent about transition** to adult gastroenterology.

The next problem is **delayed puberty and small stature**. Tom's voice has just started to deepen. He describes a small amount of pubic and axillary hair. He is lagging behind his peers and feels embarrased when he gets changed for PE. His weight is 50 kg and his height is 157 cm, with a predicted height (from parental measurements) of 175 cm. Tom had a bone-age performed recently but is unsure of the results.

Tom's next problem is **anaemia**. He took a course of oral iron three months ago from his GP and this made his abdominal pain worse, so he stopped it. He suffers from fatigue and finds it difficult to concentrate in class. He cannot recall results from his latest blood tests.

Tom also suffers from **acne**, over his face, chest and back. It is worse on higher doses of steroids; Tom's mum is confident the acne will resolve with his raw food diet.

Medications

His **current medications** are:

- azathioprine 50–100 mg per day (depending on symptoms)
- prednisone 15 mg
- Pentasa 2 g bd
- iron ferrous sulfate (does not take).

There are no drug allergies. Tom has not been **immunised** but describes having chickenpox at the age of eight. He takes a variety of herbal and homeopathic treatments but I was not provided with this list today. Tom picks up his own prescriptions from the local pharmacy. He **takes his medication** most days of the week, reminded by an alert on his smartphone.

Developmental and Social History

Tom is the middle child, with an older sister (18) and a younger brother (12) who is the same height as him and very sporty. Both siblings are well, his sister is a 'brain box' and has just got into a nursing course at uni. He **lives with** his mum who works as a bank teller and his dad who is a builder. The **pregnancy and birth** were straightforward, and he had no health or development concerns until the age of 12.

Finances are clearly a difficult area for the family so I did not probe too far. Mum explained that the appointments with the naturopath and other alternative providers 'don't come cheap'.

HEEADSSS Assessment

Socially, Tom is in year 11, but takes year 10 classes. His best subject is maths, he trusts his teacher. He doesn't like school otherwise. He has frequent trips to the nurse's office with abdominal pain, and cannot count how many sick days he has had off school this term. He is falling behind with his school work. He admits to trying alcohol and marijuana to 'fit in'. Tom has tried smoking cigarettes a few times. He is ambivalent about the effects of smoking on his Crohn's disease, but hates being sick all the time and states that putting on a 'brave face can be hard'. Tom has two good friends, Eli and John, who are now in the year ahead of him. He does not have a girlfriend and has never been sexually active. Before he was diagnosed with Crohn's disease, Tom was a keen sportsman, doing swimming, cricket and soccer, and would like to play team sports again. He likes Xbox and has a Facebook account. He wants to learn to drive.

There is no **family history** of inflammatory bowel disease but his mum has irritable bowel syndrome.

Systems Review

Systems review was unremarkable.

Examination

On **examination**, Tom appeared younger than his age of 16 years. He had conjunctival pallor and cushingoid facies. Sparse axillary hair was noted. There was an acneiform rash over the cheeks and back, with small pustules and comedones.

The **heart rate** was 70 beats/minute and regular, the **blood pressure** was 100/70. The height and weight were as previously mentioned. Cardiovascular and respiratory examinations were unremarkable. On examination of the **abdomen**, there was a midline scar and a right upper quadrant scar consistent with previous surgery and ileostomy. The abdomen was slightly distended with generalised tenderness, but with no guarding and there was a feeling of fullness in the right iliac fossa. Bowel sounds were present. **Neurological examination** was normal. I did not examine the rectum or external genitalia.

Summary Statement

In summary, Tom is an insightful and mature 16 year old with Crohn's disease, with evidence on history and examination to suggest a current flare or partial bowel obstruction. He has not achieved his growth potential and has pubertal delay. He has symptomatic anaemia and is an occasional cigarette smoker. There is conflict within the family, and also between the family, the hospital team and his complementary medicine providers which is having a negative effect on Tom. He is facing transition of care to adult services but has little knowledge of this process. Tom states his main problem is a total lack of energy and ongoing pain, likely a combination of poorly controlled Crohn's disease and anaemia. Tom's mum states the main problem is continuing with the prednisone for long enough for the dietary changes to cure his Crohn's disease.

Problem List

There are **10 problems** which I wish to discuss.

1) Ongoing active Crohn's disease which may require surgical treatment
2) Investigation and management of anaemia
3) Ongoing management of corticosteroid treatment and side effects
4) Ongoing management of his immunosuppression, including lack of immunisation and future use of biological treatments
5) Lack of relationships with specialists and impending transition
6) Failure to thrive/growth and pubertal delay
7) Family dynamics and conflict
8) Schooling
9) Intermittent smoking
10) Management of his acne

Problem	Differential diagnosis	Investigations	Management
Ongoing active Crohn's disease with abdominal fullness and pain on examination May need surgery and is terrified of another stoma	Active Crohn's disease Infection/ collection Stricture from Crohn's disease or anastomotic stricture Tumour/mass (less likely)	Review old operative notes Review previous MRI scans and colonoscopy Arrange serological tests plus CRP, renal and liver function tests Faecal microscopy and culture to rule out infection, faecal calprotectin Restaging Crohn's disease with gastro-scopy, colonoscopy and MR enteroscopy to fully assess the extent of current disease burden No history of perianal or extraintestinal involvement but consider MRI rectum/ anal canal	Depends on investigation findings (candidate needs to think on feet) If Crohn's stricture without active disease, refer to surgeons Difficult for patient to accept, as he had a stormy course for his first operation Terrified of another stoma Mother against more surgery Needs careful discussion and meet with surgeon. Could introduce to another peer who has had surgery If active Crohn's disease, review with local prescription guidelines, maximise azathioprine and failing that, add biological therapy
Investigation and management of anaemia	Iron deficiency Vitamin B12/ folate deficiency Anaemia of chronic disease/ inflammation	FBC, blood film, iron studies, vitamin B12/ folate, thyroid function Ferritin may be falsely elevated but review inflammatory markers	Iron infusion if deficient. Oral iron is relatively contraindicated in IBD

(Continued)

(Continued)

Problem	Differential diagnosis	Investigations	Management
Management of corticosteroids	Diabetes Weight gain Acne Thin skin Osteoporosis	HbA1c measurement	Maximise azathioprine dose +/− add biological Needs prednisone sick-day-plan to avoid Addisonian crisis Bone health
Management of immuno-suppression		TPMT level and aza metabolites Full screening for biological treatment history, CXR, Quantiferon TB Gold, hepatitis/ HIV serology Serology for measles, mumps, rubella and zoster (may well have antibodies already)	Suboptimal azathioprine dose for weight and consistent dose Discuss stopping mesalazine as minimal effect on Crohn's disease plus reduces pill burden If no improvement with increased azathioprine, or depending on results of investigations, consider infliximab or adalimumab according to local guidelines Counsel Tom and his mum together and seperately regarding immunisation, explore reasons for no vaccinations in a non-judgemental way Offer annual flu vax and pneumo vax Consider HPV vax

Problem	Differential diagnosis	Investigations	Management
Lack of relationships with specialists and impending transition			Explore local guidelines for transition, and give Tom and his mum guidelines on what to expect Identify one doctor at the Royal Children's Hospital to provide continuity. Identify a specific specialist in adult services who will take his care forward Contact John the naturopath – might have other insights Encourage Tom to join local IBD support group Talk to another young person in a similar situation for peer-to-peer support
FTT/growth and pubertal delay	Endocrinological causes Nutritional compromise Effect of chronic inflammation	Vitamin D levels Review bone age to see if potential for more height (could be a motivator for Tom to agree to surgery)	Control of his disease, and surgery if indicated Dietician for calorie maximisation Difficult as mistrust and conflicting advice Consider GH Vitamin D replacement as necessary

(Continued)

(Continued)

Problem	Differential diagnosis	Investigations	Management
Family dynamics and conflict	Something else going on in family Family violence not explored today		Provide continuity with same doctors involved in his care Earn Tom's trust Explain about confidentiality Offer appointments that suit Have time in appointments with and without parents, so Tom's confidence and independence with his own health needs can improve Family meeting including dad could be illuminating. Might be another family member who can help with appointments
Schooling	May have other reason than Crohn's disease for suboptimal performance such as a learning disability		Control Crohn's disease Involve hospital school so when absent has goals to meet, support and accountability Full educational assessment, so his needs can be met and realistic goals set Meeting with school and medical team
Intermittent smoking			Crucial to offer full support to stop smoking, explore why he does it Smoking cessation treatments if appropriate

Problem	Differential diagnosis	Investigations	Management
Acne	Drug reaction		Reduce prednisone Consider topical treatment first Oral agents such as retinoic acid could be considered but need to do more research on using any additional medication with IBD

22

Past Exam Long Cases

Here are some of the remembered exam long cases from registrars over the last couple of years. Details have been changed to protect anonymity. You can see that some people remember every minute detail of the day whilst others have blanked it out.

Registrar 1

1) 70-ish-year-old man with his main problem being painful peripheral neuropathy but with SLE, GORD, diverticular disease with previous diverticulitis, mitral valve replacement, atrial fibrillation, multiple dental problems, osteoporosis secondary to steroids and bruising on steroids. Patient had very little understanding of his SLE. Also had relationship issues with his wife. Patient brought in a list of his medical problems but it didn't include SLE, I got this from the history.

2) 50-ish-year-old woman with non-Hodgkin's lymphoma with a history of Cushing's disease with bilateral adrenalectomies and was later found to have ACTH-producing carcinoid tumor in her lung. Also had macular degeneration, osteoporosis, GORD, hyperlipidaemia, previous cholecystectomy and renal calculi plus hysterectomy on HRT. Key issue for patient was her macular degeneration despite her significant co-morbidities. Examiners focused on macular degeneration and the effect of her loss of vision on the patient and family, lymphoma management, long-term steroid replacement post bilateral adrenalectomy, follow-up of ACTH-producing tumour, role of HRT, management of osteoporosis and assessment of recent chest pain and cardiovascular risk assessment.

How to Pass the RACP Written and Clinical Exams: The Insider's Guide,
Second Edition. Zoë Raos and Cheryl Johnson.
© 2017 John Wiley & Sons Ltd. Published 2017 by John Wiley & Sons Ltd.

Registrar 2

1) Type 1 diabetic with all complications and deceased donor renal and pancreatic transplant and amputation with prosthetic limb. Examiners only asked one question so thought I would score high but consensus mark was a 5. Goes to show that the long-held belief that minimal questions means high marks is not true!

2) Difficult patient who wasn't in the right state of mind for exams that day and her history was disjointed. She apologised many times! With luck and a barrage of questions, worked out that she had symptomatic pulmonary and cardiac sarcoidosis and her social issue was estrangement from her husband who was abusive and had lost trust with her doctors due to atypical side effects to almost all antiarrhythmic and rate control medications. She only wanted to talk about her AF and how hard it was to achieve rate control. I kept asking her directed questions until I stumbled onto a piece of information that with persistence and directly giving her names of possible conditions I finally came to her underlying medical problem. Whilst telling me about her multiple hospital admissions, she mentioned 'They didn't like the look of my chest X-ray and there were nodules or nodes...'. Sarcoidosis popped into my head by pure luck.

Registrar 3

Both long cases were complicated diabetes cases, one with a pancreatic and kidney transplant and the other had uninvestigated iron deficiency anaemia.

Registrar 4

1) Non-compliant and poorly controlled type 2 diabetic ex-physiotherapist who had a full house of diabetic complications. Every time I tried to ask him a question to redirect him, he would tell me 'If you don't stop interrupting me you are not going to get any information out of me!'. He checked his blood sugar at least five times during the hour, saying he was hypoglycaemic and needed to eat. I wish I had come up with a better plan to manage non-compliance prior to the exam!

2) 61-year-old gentleman still working as a shopkeeper with multiple medical problems but his main problem was a three-month history of shortness of breath. His other medical problems included diabetes for 20 years but he didn't know if it was type 1 or 2 and had all the typical complications including a left below-knee amputation. Also had an aortic valve replacement for severe AS, renal failure requiring temporary dialysis but had subsequently improved and DRESS syndrome with skin issues following vancomycin. His inactive problems were previous bowel cancer with left hemicolectomy, AF on warfarin with previous PR bleed and gout.

Registrar 5

1) 60-year-old retired male nurse with long-standing type 2 diabetes and full house of micro- and macrovascular complications. Had several foot ulcers on exam and had had a hypoglycaemic event during the previous candidate's long case. Also had severe depression with suicidal ideation, painful osteoarthritis, untreated hepatitis C, morbid obesity with previous gastric bypass and IHD. Patient required lots of interruptions to bring him back on track. Problem list included:
- management of depression
- hepatitis C
- recurring obesity post bypass and worsening OA
- management of severe OA pain
- management of diabetes.

Examiners asked questions about management of his obesity, explain why his HbA1c had reduced recently with increase in hypoglycaemic events, treatment of hepatitis C and management of foot ulcers.

2) 69-year-old retired community constable with AF, IHD, type 2 diabetes, ESRF and recent GI bleed of unclear cause. Problem list included:
- worsening SOB over last two months of unclear cause – examiners asked for differential diagnosis which included fast AF, CHF, COPD as ex-smoker, asbestos exposure, anaemia following recent GI bleed, lung cancer
- mobility following debridement of leg ulcers, using crutches but had difficulty getting around house
- investigation of GI bleed.

I forgot to check his gait and ask for vaccination history and relationship with GP which examiners asked me about! I passed, though.

Registrar 6

1) Middle-aged man with recurrent renal transplant for FSGS. He was a little depressed and had post-transplant diabetes. Also had moderate asymptomatic AR.
2) Middle-aged lady with diffuse scleroderma. She had had multiple previous admissions with severe multiorgan involvement but was stable currently. She was also being investigated for faecal incontinence. She had a lot of social problems including financial issues, teenage children with disability who lived at home and husband with recent psychological problems and being made redundant.

Registrar 7

1) Diabetes and difficult-to-control hypertension in a very well man. Patient was very knowledgeable and compliant. Did not have significant end-organ damage.
2) Young guy with second renal transplant. He also had a child with severe autism. Lots of other social issues too.

Registrar 8

1) Multiple issues:
   - connective tissue disease
   - preference for alternative medications
   - steroid complications
   - functional limitations
   - mild spastic paraparesis secondary to MS
   - panhypopituitarism
   - osteoporosis
   - recurrent UTI
   - hypercholesterolaemia with cardiovascular risk factors in setting of chronic illness.
2) 48-year-old woman with vasculitis, bronchiectasis (DDx pulmonary vasculitis), coeliac disease and hypothyroidism. Main issues were:
   - vasculitis
   - shortness of breath
   - side effects of long-term steroid use
   - renal impairment

- autoimmune disease
- financial issues.

Registrar 9

1) Chronic renal disease secondary to small vessel vasculitis with vascular risk factors, medication side effects and social issues.
2) Rheumatoid arthritis with other medical problems including hypertension and chronic renal disease.

Registrar 10

1) Type 1 diabetes with recurrent hypoglycaemic episodes and depression in an elderly woman with RA.
2) Renal transplant in a patient who didn't know he had AF and was on warfarin. May have had some cognitive impairment.

Registrar 11

1) 55yo Māori gentleman. Main issues:
   - ESRF secondary to diabetic nephropathy
     - On home haemodialysis but previously had peritoneal dialysis
     - Vascular access problems and currently with an artificial fistula
     - Infection problems with previous infected grafts and previous endocarditis
   - Diabetes
     - Microvascular complications of renal failure, retinopathy (blind in one eye and questionable whether able to drive), peripheral neuropathy
     - Macrovascular – likely cardiac disease
   - Endocarditis with resultant aortic regurgitation
   - Undiagnosed hepatomegaly
     - Likely due to heart failure and fluid overload but no other signs of overload (JVP +2 cm and no peripheral oedema)
   - Living far from hospital and couldn't drive

   Difficulty with this patient was that he had forgotten his medication list and none was provided. More difficulty getting the history and trying to get as much information from him and then a thorough examination as the examiners expected you to find the hepatomegaly. I was lucky and realised that the examiners would not expect me to get much information about his medications so I did not spend much time on this and there was enough going on to not worry about it and I passed. The other candidate spent too much time on the medications, missed the murmur and hepatomegaly and subsequently failed the case.

2) Elderly man whose main issues were:
   - Ankylosing spondylitis
     - Limited Schober's test
     - Currently on adalimumab
     - Well and asymptomatic currently
   - Syncopal events
     - Seen by a neurologist and told they were atypical migraines (but patient had no headaches)
     - Previous MRI brain normal
     - Had a murmur and previous echo was normal
   - Impotence (I missed this because I did not ask and it was the first question they asked me!)

This man was still working as a farmer and was generally well. The discussion mainly centred about his syncope management and investigation and whether he should drive. I said I would look it up in the 'Medical Aspects of Fitness to Drive'; the other candidate said he thought he could drive because a neurologist said it was only a migraine (he failed and I passed). Discussion was also around side effects of adalimumab and mainly the skin cancer risk in a farmer.

Registrar 12

1) Combined renal and pancreatic transplant on immune suppression and history of acute rejection. Also had difficult to control type 1 diabetes with associated end-stage nephropathy and post-transplant recurrent pancreatitis.

2) Cushing's syndrome and panhypopituitarism post pituitary resection. Was on hormone replacement. Also had type 2 diabetes and was a Jehovah's witness on warfarin for recurrent venous thromboembolism.

Registrar 13

1) 40-ish-year-old Caucasian lady post liver transplantation for primary biliary cirrhosis. Some social issues including limited education (left school after form 4), never married but had an adult son still living at home, had been seeing a psychologist for 20 years due to anxiety. Examiners asked me multiple times whether I knew why she left school so early and I said I didn't know. In hindsight, she may have had a learning disability or some mild form of intellectual impairment. When I asked whether she went to university or had School Certificate, she did repeatedly say she was not smart enough. She was also a bit more vague than expected for her age but she tried really hard to answer my questions. She also had no idea what this exam was about. I sat with her in the last five minutes of the exam chatting about things in general and she asked me if I was training to be a nurse.

2) Woman in early 30s with eosinophilic granulomatosis with polyangiitis (had to try very hard not to say Churg–Strauss syndrome and not to get tongue-tied during the presentation) with cardiac involvement. Diagnosis was about one year ago. Difficulty weaning down prednisone as kept having flares if prednisone reduced past 8 mg/day. Started on azathioprine six weeks prior. Some social issues including having to stop working as an occupational therapist and currently on a sickness benefit, financial difficulties but parents helping out intermittently, unable to play sport (normally plays touch rugby) but no psychological issues such as depression or anxiety. Patient was a good historian with good insight into her current illness and tried to be helpful.

Registrar 14

1) Marfan's syndrome who had cardiomyopathy on a background of aortic incompetence/aortic root dilatation requiring an AVR and Bentall's procedure. I think he had a biventricular PPM/ICD as well. Other issues were he had a daughter with marfanoid features who was being investigated. In the last 20 minutes, he also remembered to tell me he had diabetes mellitus – fortunately not overly complicated. He was very helpful and obliging with directing me to what the examiners had asked and examined. I remember feeling

aggrieved that his medication list was incomplete, missing out his warfarin and PRN frusemide although he knew he was on it when I asked him.

2) Man with idiopathic pulmonary fibrosis (although he only knew he had 'lung scarring') and lumbar spinal stenosis as well as a sensory peripheral neuropathy. He told me the examiners spent a lot of time on the sensory examination of his legs and it was only when they pushed me on it that I realised the sensory deficits were not consistent with spinal stenosis alone. They possibly thought it was alcohol related as he did have previous heavy alcohol intake and he may have had mild cognitive impairment linked in with this. He wasn't a professional patient and was prone to start rambling if you let him.

Registrar 15

1) 69-year-old female with long-standing ankylosing spondylitis and psoriatic arthritis, affecting her mobility. She was started on adalimumab a year ago and recently developed hypertension (possibly secondary to steroid use).

2) 59-year-old man with implanted PPM/ICD (had several complications from surgery) for VF/VT (had one cardiac arrest) who was also still on an 'excessive/aggressive' treatment regimen (amiodarone, flecainide, beta-blocker) which had resulted in several complications (testicular atrophy/impotence, gynaecomastia, worsening Raynaud's symptoms), all of that on the background of long-standing MCTD (mainly Raynaud's but also had scleroderma-like mouth).

Registrar 16

1) Failing cardiac transplant with valvulopathy. Struggled to find things to discuss as was a bit out of my depth and the main issue was whether he was a candidate for a repeat transplant. Examiners talked about azathioprine metabolism and gout with me, as they said they didn't want to talk about areas none of us knew anything about!

2) Bilateral lung transplant (two transplants in one day!) for primary pulmonary hypertension with ethical issues around not disclosing familial component to teenaged/adult children. Lots of time spent focusing on medication side effects.

Registrar 17

1) SLE nephritis.
2) Recent viral endocarditis, hepatitis B cirrhosis, renal failure, IHD, diabetes, inguinal hernia. The patient, although charming, denied knowledge of many of his conditions and the discussion ended up focusing on whether or not he was a suitable surgical candidate for his hernia repair (which was his biggest concern).

Registrar 18

1) Liver transplant with recurrent sinus infection.
2) ESRF patient on haemodialysis with AS.

Registrar 19

1) 64-year-old female with rheumatoid arthritis, gastric bypass and undifferentiated severe back pain.
2) 83-year old female with rheumatoid arthritis, PMR, bronchiectasis, cold haemaglutinin disease +/− underlying lymphoma, CAD and ongoing angina, rotator cuff injuries with functional impairment and 20 other things medical and social!

Registrar 20

1) Granulomatosis with polyangiitis in a current inpatient with issues regarding control of type 2 diabetes secondary to prednisone use and poor insight into his disease (and insulin use) plus some other background problems also present.
2) HIV (controlled) with peripheral neuropathy, type 1 diabetes, strokes, Parkinson's-like gait, recent tachycardia of unknown cause and recent

manifestation of Raynaud's phenomenon with telangiectasia (not otherwise specified), who started bleeding spontaneously during the long case!

Registrar 21

1) Primary immunodeficiency.
2) Diabetes with complications plus upper limb neuropathy secondary to lead poisoning (worked as a painter/sander).

Registrar 22

1) Systemic sclerosis with pulmonary fibrosis.
2) Renal transplant for presumed nephrotic syndrome with new-onset diabetes after transplant and BCC resection. Examiners commented in feedback that I did not put emphasis on dietary advice and weight loss for improving glycaemic control. It does pay to go back to the basics! Despite this, I scored quite well in this case.

Registrar 23

1) 59-year-old male with Takayasu's arteritis (3 NSTEMI, 8 PCI, 2 CABG, AVR, aortic root replacement, multiple arterial thrombi, stroke) plus glucocorticoid side effects, blackouts on warfarin, sexual dysfunction and financial strain.
2) 65-year-old male with adrenomyeloneuropathy and childhood Addison's disease (impaired gait, impotence, bladder dysfunction) plus DVTs on warfarin, multifaceted high falls risk, proximal myopathy, symmetrical inflammatory small joint polyarthropathy and limited rehabilitation facilities post earthquake.

Registrar 24

1) Primary sclerosing cholangitis with obstructive jaundice requiring liver transplant with mild ulcerative colitis only and no history of cirrhotic decompensation prior to transplant. Now presents 14 years post transplant and with worsening hypertension possibly as a

complication of tacrolimus but otherwise no immunosuppressant side effects. Secondary issue of depression. Socially isolated. Did not completely fulfil DSM-IV criteria for depression although she is on an SSRI. Apparently only gone to school until aged 12, which I didn't get but she told another candidate. Talked about bowel cancer screening.

2) 21-year-old student who was diagnosed with eosinophilic granulomatosis with polyangiitis after two years of chronic cough and repeated course of antibiotics which didn't clear it. She also developed asthma-like wheeze with exacerbations during this time. In October 2012, her chest X-ray showed RUL consolidation and because it did not clear on follow-up chest X-ray and with eosinophilia (up to 2), she was diagnosed with eosinophilic granulomatosis with polyangiitis. Now controlled on a lowish dose of prednisone and sulphasalazine. Tried azathioprine but didn't work. Not tried methotrexate. Complicated by weight gain of 10 kg with moon face, buffalo hump and increased appetite but no other prednisone complications. Bone density scan done six months ago. Never sexually active so no cervical smear. Social concern of being unable to work and frustrated that she is unlike other young people. Parents live four hours drive away but supportive and fly down to support her when needed. No other connective tissue features or renal involvement. Ongoing issue of significant fatigue so unable to hold down job that required her to work on schedule, but thinking of going back to study as something to do with her time. She hadn't planned how to do that realistically in terms of finances. Forgot to ask about drinking and drug history but not smoking history and just said 'yes important things I should ask' but didn't. Also had a lack of insight into what the disease actually means and how it manifests itself.

Registrar 25

1) Systemic sclerosis with ILD and possibly pulmonary hypertension. She was taking steroids and mycophenolate. Also had a proximal myopathy. Suffering problems with family bereavement, stress around insurance claim for house flood. Case went quite well.

2) Renal transplant with metabolic complications including new-onset diabetes. The patient kept eating takeaways and putting weight on. Also had recurrent pancreatitis and BPH.

Registrar 26

1) Heart transplant for idiopathic or viral myocarditis.
2) Lung transplant for primary pulmonary hypertension.

Registrar 27

1) Elderly retired man with eosinophilic granulomatosis with poly-angiitis on long-term immunosuppression with bronchiectasis and recurrent sinus and ear infections. Also had multiple co-morbidities and also probably mildly cognitively impaired. OMG, this was an awful long case and first case of the day. He had a hearing impair-ment but couldn't wear his bilateral hearing aids because of his blocked grommets! I spoke so loudly during the history that unfor-tunately the entire outpatient department could hear me and as I got more anxious, I spoke louder and louder and faster … I was worried I was starting to scare the patient. At one stage, I did an Abbreviated Mental Test and when I said 'Who is the current prime minister?', another candidate's patient three rooms away answered 'John Key'. During the presentation, one of the examiners dozed off then the head examiner stopped me while I was talking about the medications to skip to the examination. They asked questions about immune suppression and recurrent infections and also vasculitis management and identification of active disease. The patient also told me he had reduced immunoglobulins (so I assumed this was hypogammaglobulinaemia as he had recurrent sinus/ear infections) so I also discussed differentiating secondary and primary immune deficiency for a long time. Turns out he has no immune deficiency at all (I think the patient may have just got-ten a bit confused, just like he was adamant he hadn't been on prednisone 'for years' but was on 15 mg!). I left the room and was certain I had failed but in the end I weirdly got a 6.

2) Middle-aged man with active Crohn's disease and associated anky-losing spondylitis causing social isolation, inability to work and alcohol dependence. Nice case and lots to talk about. Questions were about Crohn's management and options for him, TNF inhibi-tor indications and adverse effects. They also asked about pharma-cological management of alcohol dependence and depression and I dug myself a nice big hole. They didn't show any imaging or bloods.

Paeds Point

We have not included real-life paediatric long cases for this edition, after extensive consultation. In New Zealand, the paediatric population who come in for the exam is sparse. The logistics of selecting the right mix of patients and getting a small person and a parent to an exam centre that can be far away from home makes for a very small pool. Our paediatric advisors feel it would be unfair to exam organisers to list past patients, and we agree.

23

An Introduction to the Short Case

The short case is 15 minutes of hell. First, you're given a stem. Next, you perform a thorough and systematised physical examination individualised to the case. You then summarise your findings, which is closely followed by grilling from the examiners, including lots of questions and investigation results being thrown at you from all sides. The alleged similarity of short cases to medical school OSCEs can lull the unsuspecting candidate into a false sense of security, some believing that reading Talley and O'Connor the week before the exam will be enough – if only! Passing a short case takes practice, and is in a different stratosphere to the standard expected from medical students. Long cases induce more fear, so some candidates leave short case preparation too late. Forty percent of your total grade will come from short cases, so we strongly suggest getting stuck into short and long cases equally.

Short case preparation helps you swiftly examine patients, think on your feet and come up with sensible investigation strategies, which is excellent prep work for your long cases.

Stem 1 minute	Doing the examination 6–8 minutes	Summary statement 1–2 minutes	Management plan 3–4 minutes	Grilling session 4–7 minutes

Marking Schedule for the Short Case

You will be marked on your examination technique, your ability to get the diagnosis and discuss the patient afterwards. On page 219 is an adapted version of the RACP marking schedule. You will become frustrated with 'yeah, that was an OK short case, probably a pass' as

How to Pass the RACP Written and Clinical Exams: The Insider's Guide, Second Edition. Zoë Raos and Cheryl Johnson.
© 2017 John Wiley & Sons Ltd. Published 2017 by John Wiley & Sons Ltd.

feedback. It will help you greatly if your practice examiners mark you against this schedule, so you know when you are approaching the expected standard (see Chapter 31 for advice on giving and receiving feedback). This way, you will know your areas of difficulty and can fix these constructively. Just like in your long cases, expect your first month of short cases to grovel in the 2s and 3s.

In the long case, you need to be **in touch with the real world** but for the short case, you need to **put on a show**. Think of yourself as an actor, learning lines and witty repartee as best you can, then being thrown into an impromptu theatre-sports situation. The more preparation you do beforehand, the more likely you are to be able to cope with whacky cases thrown at you on the day. We have all moaned and groaned about the short cases and said things like, 'It's an artificial situation; who purely examines patients without taking a history first, how archaic'. That's all true but there are situations where a physician has to rely heavily on his or her skills of observation and examination, such as:

- the confused patient
- the patient who doesn't know why they've been referred to clinic
- when you don't speak the patient's language
- the screening exam (which often throws up unexpected murmurs).

Paeds Point
We realise you often can't get any history from your little patients and have to rely heavily on physical examination, smarts and acute skills of observation on a daily basis. We could learn a lot from you.

Points to Prove in the Short Case

- Showing compassion.
- Excellent bedside manner.
- Having a slick, practised, polished examination style.
- Presenting your findings in a logical, succinct and confident manner.
- Synthesising your findings to the most likely diagnosis.
- Offering a considered differential diagnosis.
- Asking for appropriate investigations.
- Interpreting those investigations.
- Offering treatment/management options for this patient.
- NOT making up signs.

Marking schedule for short cases.

Mark	Approach	Technique	Accuracy	Interpretation of signs	Investigations
1	Inappropriate, rude and insensitive	Unable to complete an appropriate examination	Missed everything	No diagnosis made. Unable to respond to any prompting	Unable to suggest reasonable investigations and misinterprets or fudges what is given
2	Hurt the patient, examiners had to step in to prevent more pain	Didn't finish in time Needed substantial examiner intervention.	Missed major signs and found signs that were not there (fibbed and fudged)	Unable to suggest diagnosis, goes down the wrong track, life-lines not taken	Unable to use investigations to assist in diagnosis Inappropriate dependence on investigations
3	Hurt the patient but figured it out and tried to make amends	Needed prompting to proceed with examination	Missed some major signs, found some major signs, didn't include important negatives	Difficulty interpreting signs More than minor prompting but recognised life-lines Differential diagnosis scanty	Needs prompting to receive investigations Some correct interpretation When given investigations, complains about quality
4	Introduces self Respectful of modesty and of discomfort Did not hurt the patient	Good, confident examination, in time frame, fluent technique Can think on feet and adapt the exam according to signs found	Found all major signs, including significant negatives	Appropriate interpretation of signs Formulates a reasonable and sensible diagnosis Gives a good differential diagnosis. A little prompting OK	Asks for the correct investigations results, interprets correctly and relates back to the patient's findings Minor prompting is OK in a complex case

Mark	Approach	Technique	Accuracy	Interpretation of signs	Investigations
5	As above	As above with flair	Found major and minor signs, including relevant negatives	Identifies most likely diagnosis, justifies it and a sensible differential diagnosis list	Correctly interprets all major findings as above
6	As above	As above, with flair and finesse	As above, but slick and mature	As above, with an excellent differential	As above, and can integrate with findings with insightfulness and no need for prompting
7	As above	As above, asked to take over as examiner	Found everything the examiners did, perhaps more	Nails it Discusses alternative diagnoses and pitfalls therein at a consultant level	Thorough, integrated approach and understands subtleties Recognises areas of doubt, performing at a consultant level

Summary

- A short case is 15 minutes long but there is a lot to cover – greeting the patient/examiners, doing a thorough examination, presenting a summary and enduring a grilling.
- Short cases = 40% of your total clinical exam mark. Underestimate them at your peril!
- It takes a lot of practice to get really slick with your short cases, and practice takes time. Start early.
- Resign yourself to the chore of short case preparation. Get your study group all fired up – you are going to need each other!

24

How to Put On a Show

Now you know the basics of short cases, it is time to get to grips with specifics. The short case is a play of three parts: first, you have to do the '**Examination Routine**', next a '**Presentation Speech**' and finally a '**Thinking on your Feet**' display during question time as you dodge questions about investigations and patient management.

Part 1: Examination Routine – How to Practise

What is the Method for Examining Patients in a Short Case?

Use what your examiners use, and let Talley and O'Connor (or *Examination Paediatrics*) be your guide. Now is not the time for inventing a new way of examining the abdomen. Check with someone senior that your method isn't too way-out and then practise, practise, practise until each short case routine is permanently etched into your brainstem. Why the brainstem? Well, on the day (unless you are supremely confident), your cerebral cortex will turn to mush and be no help at all. Then your frontal lobe will decompensate in sympathy. Your lizard-brain needs to fire up and this only comes with a lot of practice. You need to be interpreting the signs as you go, not trying to remember what comes after checking for clubbing.

Who Should I Practise On?

- **Step 1: Healthy volunteers**. This is particularly helpful in getting the order right for exams like thyroid and 'speech' exams. Make use of anyone you live with and study group friends. Only when you can

How to Pass the RACP Written and Clinical Exams: The Insider's Guide, Second Edition. Zoë Raos and Cheryl Johnson.
© 2017 John Wiley & Sons Ltd. Published 2017 by John Wiley & Sons Ltd.

give your partner/mum/neighbour a cardiovascular exam in seven minutes in your sleep should you move on to ...

- **Step 2: Your current batch of inpatients or clinic patients**. Your house officer might groan but in your daily work, pick a system for each patient and do one short case exam routine on each, timing yourself to seven minutes. It doesn't matter if there are no signs. Nail the routine down pat.
- **Step 3: Real patients with reliable signs** – patients that you've not met, who are examined by you and with a practice examiner present, under exam conditions. More on this shortly. You may be tempted to jump straight to this step. We do not recommend this. Performing the routine *and* finding signs under exam conditions takes practice.

How Long Should I Take for Each Practice Short Case with a Real Patient?

Allow 15 minutes to get through the examination for the first week as you get used to remembering the routine and finding signs at the same time. Your ultimate goal is to get through a non-neurological short case exam in seven minutes and a neurological exam in eight minutes. At the beginning, when you are practising short cases, the practice examiner should warn you at six minutes. Closer to the exam, leave out this cue because no one warns you on the day.

How Do I Find These Real Patients?

You knew this was coming. Remember? You saw us trawling around the wards, cap in hand pleading 'Short cases for the poor registrars? Anyone with good signs, murmurs, crackles, anything?'. It was a total mission then, and it still is! Each hospital has a slightly different system for collecting cases. Whatever the system, it needs to respect patient privacy and confidentiality. Ensure you share the details of patients who are willing to be practised upon with your colleagues. You will gain nothing but enemies in high and low places by hiding details of patients. Passing and failing on the day is entirely dependent on individual performance – unlike the written exam, no computer or actuarial equation is involved.

We mainly practised on inpatients and would regularly call the subspecialty registrars to see if they had suitable cases. We travelled to different hospitals at the weekends, swapping details of suitable and willing cases between ourselves. It is difficult to organise outpatient short cases outside a mock exam. As we discussed right at the start, if you have a particular knowledge or clinical experience gap, it is worth your while spending half a day in a specialty clinic to get your head around this area.

The cold harsh reality of trying to practise is thus:

- It takes 30–45 minutes to do one (yes, one) practice short case with one candidate, including the examination, presentation and discussion.
- It takes another 15 minutes to drag yourself to the next ward.
- If there are two of you, you will see two short cases each; this will take about four hours and you'll be exhausted afterwards. You'll probably need a cup of tea at some point too.

A Few Tricks of the Trade

- Send your most charming study groupie to ask the patient nicely.
- Explain you are fully qualified doctors studying to be specialists.
- Thank the patient before and afterwards.
- Making the patient a nice cup of tea (as long as not NBM) is a nice touch.
- If they say no, leave them alone. Tell others to leave them alone too.
- Weekend mornings are the optimal time for study group short cases, with less competition for the patient's time and a lower likelihood of visitors. Organised sessions have to fit in with your practice examiners.

Routines to Have Down Pat

These are some of the examination routines that you may be given on the day:

- Cardiovascular
- Respiratory
- Abdomen/gastrointestinal/haematological
- Upper limb neurology
- Lower limb neurology
- Cranial nerves
- Gait and proceed (Parkinson's disease, spastic gait, foot drop, cerebellar)

- Eyes and proceed (visual field defect, thyroid, cerebellar)
- Speech and proceed (dysarthria, expressive dysphasia)
- Hands and proceed (small joint arthropathy, scleroderma)
- Specialised endocrine (Cushing's, acromegaly, hypertension, thyroid)
- Random stuff where no amount of preparation will help ('This patient has had an operation, please proceed' is a good example)

It is a general 'rule' that, on the day, you should have at least one cardiovascular exam and one neurological exam. The other two could be anything.

It is well beyond the scope of this book to describe how to do each of the short case routines listed above. This is expertly explained by Talley and O'Connor, Ryder and other excellent resources. Everyone has a slightly different examination technique but do not deviate too far or you will confuse the examiners. It is really important to stick to your routine so your brainstem can take over on exam Day. It is not cool to break from convention completely, such as doing the cranial nerves in alphabetical, rather than numerical order.

General Pointers for a Good Routine

Examining a patient in a short case is one part 'getting the signs' and one part 'being seen to get the signs'. You may quickly do some percussion and be convinced there is no dullness present, but unless the examiner saw that percussion, you won't get the mark for it. This means your examination performance takes on a show-like quality. Every action is made bigger and more obvious for the audience's benefit. At times, it may feel like you are some sort of glamour model on a game show demonstrating wasting of a calf muscle, but this overacting is worth it. You'll probably find that you aren't hamming it up too much, you are just making it obvious you are 'observing the patient', not staring blankly into space.

For all the examination routines, make sure that you cover the following areas.

- Demonstrate that those signs that support the diagnosis are present: 'Oh look, there is a constricted pupil'.
- Demonstrate that signs that would support another diagnosis are absent: 'But wait, there is no ptosis'.

- Show that you know that the disease affects more than one organ system: 'Look at me; I know that rheumatoid arthritis can affect the lungs'.
- Show that you know that treatments can cause signs too: 'Gosh, that looks like a cushingoid face from steroid treatment'.

Examiners mark you on your attitude and approach to the patient so this is an important thing to pay attention to. Make sure that the patient is adequately exposed but exposure to the point of hypothermia is not appropriate. Likewise, make sure that the patient is seated comfortably in the bed with the pillow appropriately positioned. Be careful during palpation … think firm but gentle, not rugby prop!

Conversely, examiners often point out that patients are not made of glass and won't break if you ask them to raise their arms. If performing asterixis during the respiratory exam, ask the patient if they have wrist pain before doing the test but palpation of the wrists wastes time. Same goes for the shoulder when testing for a waterhammer pulse.

Cardiovascular Routine Tips and Pitfalls

You can count on getting at least one CVS exam in your short cases. They are considered the 'bread and butter' of medicine so you are expected to completely nail an aortic stenosis case.

- Remember to look for a malar rash while you are observing.
- Don't ask what the blood pressure is, just get on and do it. Lying and standing. Left arm and right arm. We all know that nurses kindly do blood pressures for us most of the time; consequently, some doctors really muck this up when left to their own devices. On the day, and in your practice sessions, it is reasonable of the examiners to move you on from the blood pressure. Sometimes the only finding is a blood pressure differential.
- Don't forget to look for a mitral valvotomy scar – usually well hidden by the left breast.
- Remember to reposition the patient to enhance the murmurs.
- Do dynamic and respiratory manoeuvres to bring out the murmur even more. Practise how you are going to tell the patient to do the Valsalva!
- Do a hepatojugular reflex because it's quite a reliable sign.
- Don't put too much faith in a carotid bruit being there or not.

- If you think you have found aortic incompetence or mitral valve prolapse, go back and quickly see if there is anything to suggest Marfan's syndrome.

Respiratory Routine Tips and Pitfalls

- Formally count the respiratory rate rather than just saying the patient is tachypnoeic.
- Look or ask for the sputum pot as the examiners may have planted one.
- Look for steroid skin changes, interscapular fat pads and cushingoid facies.
- Look for Horner's syndrome if there is evidence of T1 wasting.
- Forced expiratory time is a good indication of air trapping.
- Look carefully for a pneumonectomy scar and little radiation tattoos.
- Tactile fremitus is notoriously unreliable so don't hang your hat on this finding.
- If there are crackles, make sure you get the patient to cough so you can see if they clear.
- Go to the patient's back first, then examine the anterior chest. Signs are usually more apparent posteriorly.
- Make sure the patient is comfortable bent in half while you examine their are spending time listening to their chest – ask them to put their legs over the side of the bed.

Abdominal Routine Tips and Pitfalls

- Percuss the spleen before palpating it. Saves time and prodding!
- Know how to tell the difference between a spleen and a kidney.
- Decide whether this is a gastroenterological or haematological cause of hepatosplenomegaly by looking for peripheral stigmata.
- If you decide it's a gastro case, look carefully for signs of hepatic decompensation, and clues for an underlying cause (tattoos for hepatitis C being the obvious).
- If you decide it's haem, look for lymphadenopathy, Port-a-Caths and radiation tattoos.
- Don't forget to listen for renal bruits and feel for an AAA.
- Always mention that you would like to complete the exam with a PR and examination of the external genitalia.

Oh wow, how we dreaded neurology short cases. Neuro is something most candidates have little exposure to. The only answer is to follow our steps, get the exam technique sorted on normal volunteers, then practise on as many patients as you can who have abnormal signs.

- The neurological examinations must be embedded in your brainstem by practising on people with and without signs again and again. And again.
- Be prepared to be asked 'Where is the lesion?'. Even if you don't know what the diagnosis is, you should be able to logically narrow it down to where it is. To put this extremely simply, think from the top down (cerebral hemispheres, brainstem, spinal cord, nerve root, nerve plexus, peripheral nerve, neuromuscular junction, muscle).
- Make sure you can confidently tell the difference between UMN signs and LMN signs.
- Make sure you can discriminate between neuropathy and myopathy – another favourite.
- Make use of the gait exam at the beginning of a lower limb exam; it gives you a chance to observe and think. In the upper limbs, use pronator drift as a screen before you start.
- Use the examiners to help 'supervise' the patient walking. This way you are seen to be patient-safety savvy and you won't run the risk of having to catch a patient on your own. Proper assessment of the gait requires you to stand back and observe. Don't forget about the walking aid!
- If there are lower limb signs, then check the back for signs of trauma, scars and radiation marks.
- Mention you would want to ask the patient about bladder and bowel function, if this is relevant.
- Co-ordination is unreliable in the presence of weakness so don't get too excited.
- Tailor the routine to the stem you have been given. If they mention speech, then skip the eyes but make sure you test swallowing, writing and reading.
- Leave the sensory exam till last because even neurologists will tell you that it is subjective and confusing.

> **Paeds Point**
>
> Be prepared for anything! Along with congenital and rheumatic heart disease, CF, bronchiectasis and liver disease you might see:
> - Short stature, tall stature
> - Big head, little head
> - Dysmorphic child
> - Floppy baby
> - Gait
> - Complications of prematurity.
>
> Just as outlined for the adult patients, have a default routine for every short case you do:
> - Introduce yourself to the patient and parent/carer.
> - Wash or gel your hands.
> - Repeat the stem out loud or in your head.
> - Look around the room for clues, equipment, walkers, wheelchairs.
> - Have a general look at the child, growth and dysmorphic features.
>
> Tips for surviving:
> - Expose adequately but tactfully.
> - Involve the parent.
> - Be nice to the child, deploy toys from kit bag if needed. If you hurt or upset the child you will fail.
> - For developmental cases, present findings as you go (see page 144).

Part 2: Presenting a Short Case

Well done. You have completed your examination in the allotted seven minutes, and managed to remember all 12 cranial nerves. Now you need to put your hands behind your back, forget the patient is there, look the examiner in the eye and confidently explain your findings. This is not the time for an interpretive dance routine; keep your hands still! It is distracting to watch a candidate talk with their hands and an absolute disaster to demonstrate signs on your own body or the patient's. During the exam, the Presentation Speech and Thinking on your Feet Display will be in front of the patient. In your practice sessions, step outside the room and present your findings in a quiet place, respecting the patient's confidentiality.

For learning how to present a short case, you can't go past the MRCP books. Ryder has 'records', i.e. what you need say when formally presenting a patient with severe AS. One of the charming things about antipodeans is our casual language and relaxed approach. This does us no favours for the Clinical Exam, especially the short cases. Once again, thank the Brits. While Ryder doesn't go into a lot of detail about treatment options, it does strongly encourage a succinct and snappy presentation style (as opposed to the rambling, incoherent, waffling approach that we all started with).

For the vast majority of short cases, candidates complete their examination then summarise their findings. Exceptions include the paediatric developmental short case and a complex rheumatological case with multiple joint involvement. If you are going to 'present as you go', you need to tell the examiners and seek approval.

There are two ways of presenting your short case: the high road and the low road.

Taking the High Road

Hmm, the high-risk strategy.

> '… Thank you for asking me to see Mrs L, who has severe mitral stenosis most likely due to rheumatic valvular disease, as evidenced by …'

The candidate spits out the diagnosis in a confident fashion, and then describes the examination findings consistent with the presumed diagnosis. It is a gamble, as you have painted yourself into a corner if you're wrong. We weren't brave enough on the day, but some are. Practise this a few times beforehand, you'll see that it's quite a challenge. Most of us abandoned the high road for …

The Low Road

Welcome back to Earth. Most people would present a short case in the order in which they examined the case, screening out irrelevant rubbish and emphasising the key negative and positive findings. You can still completely nail a short case on the low road and get great marks.

Introduction:	'Thanks for asking me to see Mrs L.'
Repeat the stem:	'Her GP noticed a heart murmur, and I was asked to examine her cardiovascular system.'
Describe your findings in order:	'Mrs L was lying comfortably at rest. Her pulse was 70 beats per minute, clinically in atrial fibrillation but of normal character. The blood pressure was 130/80. Her cheeks were flushed, but there were no peripheral stigmata of infective endocarditis. There was a tapping apex beat in the 5th intercostal space, with no heaves or thrills. The heart sounds were dual, with a soft diastolic murmur best heard in the mitral area. This was loudest on expiration, and did not change with the Valsalva manoeuvre. There was no evidence of overt left or right ventricular failure.'
Say what you think:	'These findings are in keeping with moderate mitral stenosis.'
Give yourself a life-line:	'But there are other diagnostic possibilities for a diastolic murmur ...'

Short and Snappy

Keep your case presentation short and snappy at this point. No one wants to hear a long list of irrelevant negatives (the absence of clubbing, splinters, HPOA, pulsus paradoxus, jaundice, pale conjunctiva ... yawn). If you have done your acting well, it will be obvious that you looked for clubbing without you having to say that it wasn't there.

However, it is important to list the *relevant* negatives in the exam. These stand out all the more by you emphasising fewer of them in your summary. If in doubt, ask yourself the importance of a sign's presence or absence (e.g. absence of a P2 or RV heave tells you and the examiner about the absence of pulmonary hypertension in a patient with TR or lung disease).

Make sure that you mention important clinical findings (especially in your end-of-the-bed-o-gram), even if they are not related directly to the examination you have been asked to do. You look silly if you fall over the low walking frame when you approach the patient. Don't forget to mention an above-knee amputation during an abdominal short case. Look at the Medic-Alert bracelet as you never know what gems might be underneath (ask the examiners first!), and take careful note of the surroundings.

Paeds Point
All of the above applies to you too. State the obvious. Summarise rather than repeat, and please be tactful when speaking about a baby or child. There is an art to describing dysmorphic features accurately and in an orderly way without being an insensitive buffoon. Buffoons tend to fail.

Part 3: The Short Case Discussion (Grilling)

After announcing their diagnosis, many candidates stop talking. Big mistake. You are now wide open to being asked any number of nasty questions. Even worse, they may not ask you any questions and then you've missed your chance to prove what you know. We recommend that, in the exam, you keep talking until someone interrupts you. The show is not over yet!

To continue our presentation above …

Differential diagnosis:	'…which include aortic regurgitation. I note that the murmur was in mid-diastole and not early diastole and there were no other murmurs audible in the aortic region…'
Investigations:	'I would like to investigate this with…' See below for a suggested order. Discuss examinations in an orderly way, showing the examiner you are a sensible practitioner of medicine who won't jump straight to a cardiac MRI without asking for an ECG first. Also make sure that you know *why* you want that particular test and what information you want to glean from it.

At any point in your investigation discussion, the examiners will thrust papers or PowerPoint slides under your nose and wait expectantly for your brisk interpretation. Interpret, then get straight back on track. Are you now seeing how short case prep will help with your long cases too?

What Kinds of Investigations Might I Interpret on Exam Day?

- Chest or joint X-ray
- ECG
- Pulmonary function tests or spirometry (know the difference between these two!)
- Arterial blood gas

- Blood tests including hepatitis serology, rheumatological antibody tests
- HRCT lung (stick to broad terms like 'fibrosis', 'ground glass' and 'honeycombing' if it's big enough for a bee to get in there!)
- Echocardiogram

Keep it simple! Say what you see, even if it doesn't quite fit with the patient's physical findings. Be prepared to amend or modify your diagnosis based on the investigations as the examiners may have just thrown you a life-line! Calmly describe what you see and show why this doesn't fit with your earlier findings. Say that you would want to go back and re-examine the patient to confirm your findings. They may just let you.

Don't complain about the quality of an X-ray or scan. Yes, we all know that a 3×4 cm photocopied image is less than ideal but no one likes a whinger, and you will lose the benefit of the doubt of the examiner, which is a half-mark, and that can be the difference between passing and failing. Do your best with what you are given.

When you are taking someone through a short case, imagine you are an examiner. Throw them an ECG or X-ray and ask for an interpretation. Ask them for a differential diagnosis. Test their confidence. Interrupt mid-sentence.

Firstly, I would take a full history and complete a full examination of the patient, including (if relevant) the rectum and external genitalia.

	I would take a history, including:	Basic tests I would like to start with:	Specialised tests I would consider would be *(pick what is relevant for your case)*:
CVS	• IHD risk factors • Angina • Exercise tolerance • CHF symptoms • Childhood illness • IVDU	• ECG • CXR • FBC • U&E • Urine dipstick • Two sets of blood cultures	• Cardiac stress test • Echocardiogram • MRI • Angiography
Respiratory	• Smoking history • Occupational exposure • TB exposure • Exercise tolerance	• CXR • Spirometry • ECG • FBC • U&E • Sputum specimen (culture/cytology)	• Pulmonary function tests • HRCT • Bronchoscopy • Induced sputum • Lung biopsy

	History	Basic tests	Specialised tests
Abdominal	• Alcohol history • Viral exposure • Drug history (prescription, over the counter) • IVDU • Bowel habit • Pain • Extraintestinal symptoms • Surgical history	• AXR • FBC • Blood film • U&E • LFT • Coagulation screen • Full liver screen (hepatitis serology, autoimmune screen, iron studies, etc.) • Stool specimens (microscopy, calprotectin, fat, pancreatic elastase)	• Liver USS • Liver biopsy • ERCP/MRCP • Endoscopy (upper, lower) plus histology • Cross-sectional abdominal imaging (CT, MR) • Examination of the small bowel (enteroclysis, capsule, enteroscopy)
Haematology	• B-symptoms • Swellings • Infections	• FBC including blood film and flow cytometry • Coagulation screen • Full anaemia screen if appropriate • Other tests (JAK-2, B2MG, electrophoresis, Ig's, SFLC)	• Node FNA/biopsy • Bone marrow aspirate and trephine
Neurology	• Onset and tempo of symptoms • Continence • Alcohol history	• FBC • U&E • Thyroid function • B12, folate • Other peripheral neuropathy testing (electrophoresis, rheum screen, HIV) • Lumbar spine XR	• MRI • Nerve conduction studies • CSF examination • *Campylobacter* serology • Advanced serology testing (AChR or NMDA antibodies, etc.)
Endocrinology	• Heat/cold intolerance • Sexual function	• Urinary microalbumin • TFTs • Morning cortisol • IGF-1 • HbA1c	• Synacthen test • MRI brain

Is the Examiner Trying to Trick You?

During the discussion, you will hear examiners say things like: 'Are you sure that this woman has a lower motor neurone lesion?'. Are they testing your mettle or throwing you a life-line?

In nine out of 10 cases, the examiner is trying to save you. However, they may also be testing your confidence and ability to cope with other possibilities (a real MRCP trait). This is a delicate judgement call.

Overall, candidates who appear stubborn, openly disagree with examiners and refuse to change their mind risk failing the case. It is not because the candidate is wrong but because it's not 'physician-ly' to be argumentative and arrogant. Be prepared to be open to other possibilities in a confident, congenial manner.

> 'Well, the slow rising pulse and nature of the murmur seem to be in keeping with aortic stenosis, but this systolic murmur could arise from aortic sclerosis, the mitral valve or indeed another cardiac lesion.'

You can 'build in' a way out for yourself during your presentation if you aren't sure what the correct diagnosis is:

> 'This patient has a symmetrical, deforming polyarthritis most consistent with rheumatoid arthritis. However, there are some features that would be more in keeping with psoriatic arthritis…'

They may ask, 'So, what is consistent with psoriatic arthritis in this case?'. Take a deep breath. They just threw you a life-line.

So What is a Life-Line and How Do You Recognise One?

It may surprise you to know that the examiners actually want you to pass and want you to showcase your knowledge. Examiners do not take great delight in failing a candidate. Hence the life-line. If you see it, grab it with both hands. The bitter irony is, the more nervous the candidate, the more they are drowning in misery and the less likely that they will be able to recognise, let alone grab the life-line.

Sometimes examiners can be subtle with their life-lines but some examples include the following.

- 'Does that support your diagnosis?'
- 'Is that what you would expect to see?'
- 'Did you consider ...?'
- 'Are you sure?'

Summary

- The short case is a show of three parts: demonstrating an exam routine (including finding the signs), giving a summary of your findings and presenting a management plan while receiving a grilling from the examiners.
- Have your textbooks on hand when practising short cases and grill each other with tricky questions.
- We recommend avoiding the high road and opting for the low road in your discussion.
- Look out for life-lines, on Exam Day and also in your practice sessions.

25

Short Case Advice from Registrars

- **Don't just do something, stand there!** Do not underestimate how useful it is to stand back and repeat the stem to yourself in your mind and give yourself a few seconds to think about what you are about to do.
- **The end-of-the-bed-o-gram.** This is an underrated minute of silence. Cachexia and breathlessness at rest are unmissable signs if you stop and look for them.
- **Look around the room.** It can be a gold mine. A wheelchair, ankle foot orthoses, inhalers, GTN spray, sputum pots all give you essential information.
- For Pete's sake, **remember the stem.** Stop smirking, sonny, this is harder than it sounds. Burn it in your mind.
- **Listen carefully** when the examiner asks you what system to examine. Again, stop laughing; we have all experienced being halfway through a respiratory exam before realising … this is a gastro exam, you fool!
- Try to **remember the patient's name and age.** On the day, there are supposed to be name labels, but this can be variable. Use your two-minute stem time to memorise the patient's details along with the stem. Otherwise, statements like 'This good man' or 'this young child' will suffice. Try and act like you haven't forgotten the name even if you have. Beware of using 'elderly patient' unless the patient looks over 80 years. It's not a great look to insult your middle-aged patients by calling them old!
- Sometimes it pays not to be too specific about signs if you aren't entirely sure what's going on. Better to leave them out if you aren't sure if they were really there. Examiners, like lions on the savannah,

How to Pass the RACP Written and Clinical Exams: The Insider's Guide,
Second Edition. Zoë Raos and Cheryl Johnson.
© 2017 John Wiley & Sons Ltd. Published 2017 by John Wiley & Sons Ltd.

like nothing more than leaping on the weakest gazelle, which is how you appear if you waffle.

- **Keep talking and talking and talk 'till you can't talk no more.** This sounds like madness but you must practise talking and not stopping. Once you've presented your findings, and what you think the problem is, **don't wait to be asked a question – keep talking.** Question time risks them taking you somewhere you don't want to go; you will end up standing there blankly, looking clueless. If *you* lead the discussion, you are more likely to cover ground that you *do* know about and then you will sound smarter.
- **Ideas for discussion time.** Discuss a differential. Mention you'd like to take a full history and complete your examination. Ask for simple investigations and mention which is your investigation of choice and why. **Then keep talking!** What treatment you'd like, what complications could occur, etc.
- Of course, if the examiners interrupt, you can probably stop talking long enough to listen.
- **Don't despair if you forget to do something.** Calmly say that you would like to complete your examination by looking at the temperature chart, urine analysis … oh, and by auscultating the chest too.
- **Don't be put off if they interrupt.** This just means that you have proved that point and they want to move onto the next hurdle so they can test what else you know.
- **Expect to be pushed until you don't know the answer.** They just want to find your limits so don't be surprised if the questions get harder. It's OK to say you don't know (much better than guessing).
- It's surprising how many short cases are passed even though the candidate didn't hear the murmur, missed out parts of the exam or admitted that they didn't know how to treat myeloproliferative disease. Even if it's going absolutely appallingly, it's better to keep on trying because you may get another mark or two for sheer effort (and those two marks could make all the difference!). No short case should ever be given up for dead. **Never, ever give up.**
- When the examiner asks you a question, **close your mouth, engage your brain and then answer the question**. Don't blurt out the first thing that comes into your brain because it may not be the most appropriate answer.
- Practise short cases with **different people** and take along a text book for question time.

- Grill each other on **severity criteria for valve disease** and practise more than just AS/MR. Trawl the wards for complicated multiple valve disease or even rarer things. Candidates have also been faced with aortic coarctation, PDA and VSD on Exam Day.
- **Practise respiratory cases** with all the bells and whistles because it is actually quite a nice exam.
- Learn to do a **four-min neuro exam** on your normal buddies to allow you time to find the pathology on the real patients!
- Try to find patients to practise the **less common exams** on – neck/endocrinology/hands (rather than endless respiratory/AS/MR/stroke/neurology exams).

26

Past Exam Short Cases

The short case patients are often people who have very stable signs and get pulled in year after year. Keep that in mind when you search for practice cases in an acute hospital – that great case of crashing pulmonary oedema is probably not going to be there in the exam (at least not intentionally!).

Here are some cases from registrars who have sat the exam in the past few years. Keep in mind that the examiners don't tell you at the end if you were right or wrong, so the diagnoses may not actually be correct!

Registrar 1

1) Scleroderma. Stem was: 'This patient has been breathless, examine hands and proceed.'
2) Significant aortic regurgitation, couldn't hear a systolic murmur.
3) Neurology case with mixed UMN and cerebellar signs. I thought it was MS and the examiners seemed to encourage this line of discussion
4) ILD likely IPF.

Registrar 2

1) Examine scleroderma hands and proceed. Asked to comment on chest X-ray, ECG, ANA profile and right heart pressures on echocardiogram.

How to Pass the RACP Written and Clinical Exams: The Insider's Guide,
Second Edition. Zoë Raos and Cheryl Johnson.
© 2017 John Wiley & Sons Ltd. Published 2017 by John Wiley & Sons Ltd.

2) Respiratory exam – post lobectomy and incidental neck lump. Asked to interpret lung function tests and chest X-ray.
3) Cardiovascular exam – findings in keeping with TR. Was asked to comment on JVP waves.
4) Lower limb neurological exam – mixed sensory/motor neuropathy with foot drop and high stepping gait.

Registrar 3

1) 50-ish-year-old man presents with breathlessness on exertion and stem was: 'Examine the hands and proceed'. Man had scleroderma with multiple digital infarcts, shortened distal phalanges and tight skin over the fingers. No sclerodactyly or calcinosis. Good hand function. Proceeded to cardiorespiratory exam which was unremarkable except for a systolic murmur. No obvious signs of pulmonary fibrosis or pulmonary hypertension. Was shown a spirometry report which revealed a restrictive pattern. Total lung volume/DLCO was not given.
2) Lady presenting with exertional chest pain. I thought she had mixed aortic valve disease, however the dominant valve lesion was (I was asked what I thought the dominant lesion was) most likely aortic regurgitation based on the peripheral signs – wide pulse pressure and collapsing pulse.
3) Neurology case – not sure what it was. Caucasian woman in her 40s presenting with difficulty walking. Unable to walk on heels/toes/perform tandem gait. Rhomberg's negative. Had pes cavus which I totally forgot to mention when I was presenting my findings. Had impaired co-ordination in the right leg only. Increased tone and brisk reflexes in both legs but normal power. Possibly had patchy reduced pinprick sensation over thighs (could have been a red herring as this was subjective). No nystagmus and FNF normal. Examiners kept asking me where I thought the lesion was. I kept saying the cerebellum and spinal cord. I said the most likely diagnosis was multiple sclerosis but it could have been Friedreich's ataxia or some other hereditary ataxia. I was probably wrong. As soon as I was shown an MRI image of the brain, there was a knock on the door. The examiner said 'you ran out of time'. I felt relieved that I did not have to interpret the MRI because on a brief glance there was nothing too obvious.

4) 50-ish-year old man with shortness of breath. I thought he had idiopathic pulmonary fibrosis. Reduced chest expansion and bibasal inspiratory Velcro-like crackles. Not cyanotic and not on oxygen (no portable oxygen tank in the room). No peripheral signs suggestive of connective tissue disease. I was shown a spirometry report and CT chest image. Restrictive pattern on spirometry and CT chest showed honeycombing.

Registrar 4

1) Had neuro case that I completely bombed! Stem was: 'This man had surgery 10 years ago and since then has had difficulty walking. Examine gait and proceed'. I couldn't pick the gait but noted he had previous lumbar spinal surgery. Was expecting UMN signs instead found LMN signs and wildly inconsistent bilateral sensory signs. Babbled on about a possible UMN lesion for some reason and consequently confused myself and the examiners. Bad start to the short cases!

2) Next case was a cardiology short with HCM. Stem was palpitations in a fairly elderly woman. Apex seemed quite displaced with normal carotid pulse and the murmur didn't seem to augment with Valsalva so I wasn't confident with calling it HCM (although the fact that she knew how to Valsalva when asked should have been a giveaway). Threw in mitral regurgitation and less likely aortic stenosis. Got to see her ECG with LVH and echo with HCM, other candidates apparently didn't get up to this point so I presume I was doing OK. Got grilled on the mechanism of how the Valsalva causes HCM to augment and got saved by the bell while mumbling about SAM when asked how mitral regurgitation could be related to HCM.

3) Next short was rheumatoid arthritis with lung crackles either drug or disease related. Stem was: 'Difficulty using hands'. There was an emphasis on her neck as well and they wanted to know what I would expect to find if I thought she had atlantoaxial instability. They then produced an X-ray of her neck which I couldn't really interpret, partly due to inexperience but it was also quite poor quality so I looked at it dubiously and politely said it was difficult to interpret. They whisked it away so hopefully they agreed.

4) Final short was an elderly man with mitral regurgitation, aortic sclerosis and EF of 10–15%. Stem was something about worsening exercise tolerance. When they pushed me as to whether I thought I could hear a second murmur, I threw in the crescendo-decrescendo non-radiating murmur at the base of the heart which I initially thought was just radiation of the MR. Said it could be aortic sclerosis and was pretty stoked when the examiner informed me of the echo report later showing MR and aortic sclerosis.

Registrar 5

1) Stem – presents with abdo pain, please examine the abdomen. 60-ish-year-old female with palpable cystic mass in her abdomen and a few scars. Felt like liver as it was on the right and was also felt in the midline. Could have been a transplanted kidney that had become cystic but the scar was not the right kind of scar and the mass was not ballotable, no signs of previous fistula on her arms but could have had dialysis through tunnelled line in the past. Shown normal liver function tests. I still don't know what it was!

2) Stem – presents with shortness of breath, please examine the respiratory system. 60-ish-year-old man with ILD affecting the lower zones. Normal-looking pulmonary function tests except for DLCO of 54% which confirmed the diagnosis for me. I gave them a long list of differential diagnoses (was interrupted in the middle of the list, presumably because I was doing OK).

3) Stem – complaining of weakness, please examine the upper extremities. 20-ish-year-old man with classic myotonic dystrophy (all the features), had distal > proximal weakness, also had a high-arched palate so I spoke about association with Marfan's. His ECG and echo were normal. It was pure MD and nothing else.

4) Stem – complaining of shortness of breath, please examine cardiovascular system. 60-ish-year-old man with very faint murmur over pulmonary area. Normal echo so I said that nothing I found on cardiovascular exam could explain his shortness of breath. I was taken back to the patient and asked to look at his eyes and neck. It looked like he had irregular pupils secondary to previous surgery and features of ankylosing spondylitis. His shortness of breath must have been caused by impaired chest expansion from ankylosing spondylitis but I ran out of time to say that!

Registrar 6

1) Mixed aortic valve disease with predominant AR with hugely dilated aortic root on chest X-ray.
2) Renal transplant with polycystic kidneys but no fistula access site, only tunnel line scars. They kept asking me if I heard a murmur (which I didn't!) or if I felt an associated polycystic liver (which I didn't!).
3) ILD which looked like IPF on HRCT. Got shown pulmonary function tests and asked if I could see only one value on the test, which one would it be?
4) Neuro case – still not really sure what it was. Had severe predominantly sensory peripheral neuropathy but increased tone as well. Wondered if there were two pathologies, however examiners only wanted to talk about the peripheral neuropathy.

Registrar 7

1) Stem – examine a man with a known murmur and proceed. Dextrocardia with grade 2 AS. Even the examiners had a hard time hearing the murmur. Advice is not to panic and you will score well if you show you can modify examination appropriately even if you don't do the whole exam smoothly.
2) Stem – examine the abdomen and proceed. Chronic liver disease with all the signs of cirrhosis including spider naevi, clubbing, ascites, hepatosplenomegaly, palmar erythema, distended abdominal veins and some signs of RHF (TR murmur, raised JVP). I thought RHF was from portopulmonary hypertension but could have been cardiac cirrhosis from primary right heart pathology.
3) Stem – examine the hands and proceed. Diffuse cutaneous systemic sclerosis with all typical signs (was even given echocardiogram results to comment on after findings suggestive of ILD on respiratory exam).
4) Stem – examine gait and proceed. Cerebellar disease in 55-ish-year-old man (I still don't know the actual diagnosis but I thought it could be spinocerebellar ataxia). Likely midline cerebellar lesion since there was a full constellation of all cerebellar signs, including staccato speech and some pyramidal signs (not weakness but increased tone, some spasticity and brisk reflexes).

Registrar 8

1) Abdo case – polycystic liver disease without kidney involvement.
2) Neuro case – cerebellar signs with subtle broad-based gait and dysdiadochokinesis but normal finger-nose-finger test.
3) Cardio case – MS.
4) Resp case – differentials for LUL changes.

Registrar 9

1) Scleroderma.
2) Interstitial lung disease.
3) Aortic regurgitation.
4) Neuro case – stem was a 40-ish-year-old woman with a recent significant illness, examine her cranial nerves. She had right-sided CN III and VII involvement. All I could remember from this case was the predominant thinking process I had going on in my brain was 'Oh my goodness … what the??!!'.

Registrar 10

1) Stem – 74-year-old male with shortness of breath, examine his respiratory system. Diagnosis was chronic lung disease secondary to asbestosis, bronchiectasis and smoking with cor pulmonale. Examiners agreed signs were clubbing, increased respiratory rate, sinus rhythm, poor air entry, muscle wasting, lung crepitations and possible increased P2.
2) Stem – please examine gait and proceed. Diagnosis was cerebellar astrocytoma (posterior fossa craniectomy). Examiners agreed signs were right > left cerebellar signs, posterior fossa scar, bilateral hearing aids, VP shunt palpable and some weakness right > left.
3) Stem – Mr K has been found to have a murmur, examine his cardiovascular system. Diagnosis was MR +/- AS. Examiners agreed signs were pulse 76/min regular and bounding, BP 140/60 (wide pulse pressure), JVP 0 cm with normal wave form, apex beat displaced 2 cm lateral to MCL at 6 ICS, PSM radiating to left axilla and possibly carotids, chest clear. Showed an ECG with partial LBBB, sinus rhythm with ectopics.

4) Stem – presents with nocturia, examine abdomen and proceed. Diagnosis was renal transplant in RIF. Examiners agreed signs were two scars in RIF, transplanted kidney in RIF, no other organomegaly, soft right femoral bruit, left AV fistula, thin skin with bruising, multiple small scars on face and arms, difficult to palpate kidney in RIF secondary to overlying induration and scarring.

Registrar 11

1) Lady with chronic SOB. Thin Caucasian lady with lower lobe coarse crepitations. Diagnosis was bronchiectasis but acceptable differential diagnosis was ILD and CHF (but no other findings to support this). Shown a chest X-ray and asked what are the chest X-ray signs of bronchiectasis. Easy case.
2) 40-year-old Caucasian lady with trouble using her hands. Had mild signs of scleroderma on hands and face. Found this one hard as the signs of scleroderma were not very obvious at all.
3) 80-year-old female with no symptoms, examine her cardiovascular system. Aortic regurgitation found. Easy case.
4) 50-year-old female with recent severe illness who now has permanent facial weakness. Asked to examine cranial nerves. Signs were right sixth and seventh palsy and nystagmus. Had to also examine gait and rule out cerebellar disorder as nystagmus present. Asked what differential diagnosis was – ? pontine lesion ? post GBS. Examiners happy with 1–2 differentials.

Registrar 12

1) Abdo exam – splenomegaly (viral infection).
2) Lower limb exam – Charcot–Marie–Tooth or HSMN.
3) Respiratory exam – right apical mass.
4) Rheum exam – ankylosing spondylitis.

Registrar 13

1) Stem – this elderly lady has a cough, examine her hands and proceed. She had rheumatoid hands and basal crackles. A little tricky with the timing as unsure how quickly to move to the

respiratory exam. Had to interpret chest X-ray, lung function tests and slice of CT.

2) Myotonic dystrophy. Can't remember the stem, but if you had seen it before (you do at Tauranga Neurology Course), was pretty straightforward. Asked about type of mutation, diagnosis and management.

3) Stem – this middle-aged man is asymptomatic, examine his gastro-intestinal system. He had an AV fistula, was plethoric and had multiple abdo scars and a transplanted kidney. Was asked questions about why I thought he had CKD then lots of questions about PCKD.

4) Stem – this middle-aged woman is asymptomatic, examine her cardiovascular system. She had Marfan's, midline thoracotomy scar and a soft PSM. Question about what surgery I thought she had. I got a bit lost in the discussion talking about her murmur so didn't get far.

Registrar 14

1) Kidney transplant. Missed the fistula as it was on the other hand. Asked to examine the gastrointestinal system so took me a few minutes to get back to the kidneys.

2) Marfan's post surgery. Didn't notice any murmurs. Just called it straight away.

3) Myotonic dystrophy. They had heaps of test results I didn't ask for.

4) RA with pulmonary sequelae. They threw in the fact that she was clearly positioned for the hand exam but the stem was she was short of breath and proceed.

Registrar 15

1) Patient with dextrocardia and murmur of aortic sclerosis. Key was to think you were still on the left side. Agreed signs were low BP, JVP normal, ESM at base and no signs of CHF.

2) Stem – unsteady, examine gait and proceed. Signs were ataxic gait, past pointing, staccato speech, reduced tone, nystagmus to left,

brisk reflexes and normal power. I didn't reach diagnosis but I examined well and didn't elaborate differentials when pushed.
3) Stem – patient has cold hands, examine hands and proceed. Patient had scleroderma. Agreed signs were sclerodactyly, microstomia, crepitations in lung bases, normal P2 and normal BP.
4) Abdominal examination with hepatomegaly. Agreed signs were hepatomegaly, ascites, TR, some spider naevi, tough spleen, no lymphadenopathy, pitting oedema. Key was to pick up oedema/pulsatile liver, think TR and then examine heart.

Registrar 16

1) Interstitial lung disease.
2) Surgically repaired cervical stenosis with bilateral upper motor neurone signs in the legs.
3) Polycystic kidneys with a renal transplant and multiple skin cancers.
4) Young girl with SVC obstruction due to thrombosed Port-a-Cath. Also had unusual surgical scars and previous PEG placement. Still not sure what her underlying condition was.

Registrar 17

1) L5 radiculopathy.
2) Aortic stenosis.
3) CF with bronchiectasis.
4) Bilateral cerebellar signs with impaired vibration sensation to her head! I didn't know what was wrong with her.

Registrar 18

1) NSIP without lots of signs.
2) Severe psoriatic arthritis with cervical spine ankylosis and a neck mass.
3) Severe postural and intention tremor.
4) Severe/critical AS with a full house of signs.

Registrar 19

1) Isolated splenomegaly without any systemic signs of hepatic or haematological disease.
2) Cardiology exam – I have no idea what it actually was but I thought she had slightly dysmorphic facial features and an ejection systolic murmur which I thought may have been aortic sclerosis.
3) Proximal weakness and discussion of the differential.
4) Likely ILD with bibasal crepitations in a woman with signs of systemic sclerosis.

Registrar 20

1) Polycystic kidneys and transplant.
2) Ankylosing spondylitis.
3) Spinal cord compression.
4) Aortic regurgitation with congenital heart disease and pacemaker for heart block.

Registrar 21

1) No idea what the cardiac case was. I heard a systolic murmur and fixed splitting of S2 in a middle-aged lady with a midline sternotomy without a vein harvest scar.
2) Proximal myopathy.
3) ILD with scleroderma. I was asked to examine the patient's respiratory system. The patient had obvious sclerodactyly consistent with scleroderma so it was a matter of deciding whether it was pulmonary fibrosis or pulmonary hypertension. Since I was asked to perform a respiratory exam, I did a thorough respiratory exam and did not focus on the hands. Examiners commented on my accurate chest findings but wanted me to elaborate on the hand findings. Passed!
4) Splenomegaly. Once I made sure there was no hepatomegaly, it was a matter of showing no other signs of chronic liver disease or haematological disorders.

Registrar 22

1) Mixed AR/AS, MR and pulmonary hypertension secondary to OSA.
2) Polycystic kidneys with tender left renal transplant.
3) CIDP with concurrent spasticity.
4) ILD of UIP type with pulmonary hypertension.

Registrar 23

1) Cardio SC – feels SOB, please examine the cardiovascular system. Middle-aged woman who was very self-conscious about being undressed and two male examiners so when you attempted to expose, she tugged the gown upwards as much as she could. Not clubbed or cyanosed. Two murmurs of differing quality – one ESM and one PSM radiating to axilla. Examiner tried to suggest that MR was more of a problem but clinically no features to suggest it was severe and not in AF and no features of CHF. Chest X-ray showed normal heart. Spent too much time just discussing why I thought murmur was MR or AS. Ran out of time other than to say I ultimately wanted an echo. ECG was normal but panicked and almost overcalled LVH.

2) Rheum SC – examiner was a rheumatologist! Asked to examine the hands and proceed. I broke the bed after lying patient flat and couldn't get it back up again and special allowance was made! Skin tightening was not all that obvious but the nails were tiny wedges and the hand skin was very course. No clubbing. Fixed contracture of the wrist and positive Bower's sign. No nodules at the elbows or psoriasis evident. Mouth not obviously contracted but telangiectasia seen on the mucosa when you flip the lower lip outwards. Can't remember if the patient had fine Velcro-like crackles. No murmur. No obvious changes in the feet. I finished before the time was up and was struggling to think what else as the patient was middle aged male so was thinking anti-synthetase syndrome. Asked for autoimmune screen and then told me he was anti-Jo1 negative but ANA positive and centromere positive so told them it's limited diffuse scleroderma which is what the patient had.

3) Neuro SC – examine gait and proceed. Gait wasn't obvious and I wondered whether it was a high stepping gait bilaterally. Increased tone with hyper-reflexia and weakness on the right side more than left, upgoing plantars bilaterally, sensory deficit in glove/stocking distribution on pinprick testing, deteriorated RAM on the left worse than the right, no visual field defect, normal eye ROM with no nystagmus, speech normal and no evidence of cerebellar features. Putting it all together, I said it was most likely a demyelinating lesion, given the patient was female in 40s. Explained that I suspected to see multiple lesions and unlikely to be in the spinal cord as dissociated sensory and weakness not observed unless high in the brainstem but didn't fit with that pattern on exam. Cerebellum must have been involved due to the impaired RAMs on the left but weakness was more on the right. Sensory symptoms I thought were due to another pathology like diabetic neuropathy.

4) Respiratory SC – patient presents with a cough, please examine respiratory system and proceed. 78-year-old female with idiopathic pulmonary fibrosis. Clubbing with fine Velcro-like crackles and the trachea was central, no reduced expansion despite a thoracotomy scar. No other features to suggest arthritis. No evidence of cor pulmonale. Gave differential for crackles in the chest and ILD. Interpreted chest X-ray with increased interstitial markings. HRCT showed honeycomb with predominant basal distribution.

Registrar 24

1) Splenomegaly – I proceeded to examine for lymphadenopathy and signs of chronic liver disease of which there were none. Then I thought that patient might have PCV so I started to do a BP and look in his eyes but the examiners said this was unnecessary. Time ran out just as they were showing me his bloods.

2) Cardiac exam – difficult case. Median sternotomy scar in a 46 year old but no significant valvular disease. Turns out they had had a CABG and previous pericardial effusion but no major signs for the exam.

3) Respiratory case – CREST with ILD. Moist sounding cough so possibly some infective component as well.

4) Proximal myopathy. Stem was to examine the patient's gait and proceed. I wasted time watching him walk for ages, which was

fruitless as his gait was normal. Should have got him to squat and stand but didn't. Took a gamble and examined for weakness which there luckily was. Not enough time to do a sensory or upper limb examination so it was hard to come up with myopathy and had to be led there.

Registrar 25

1) Renal transplant and polycystic kidneys.
2) Peripheral neuropathy.
3) Aortic stenosis.
4) Interstitial fibrosis.

Registrar 26

1) Neurology – CIDP. Stem was: 'Difficulty walking, please examine the lower limbs'. Straightforward but they wanted a good differential for peripheral motor neuronopathy. I thought he had Charcot–Marie–Tooth but listed CIDP in the differential and still did fine.
2) Respiratory – thoracoplasty. Stem was: 'SOB on exertion, please examine the respiratory system'. It was a bit of a difficult exam. She had a chest wall deformity and obvious scar but the tracheal deviation was difficult to feel. She also had an odd non-mobile irregular neck mass so tried to tie it all together as a lung malignancy with upper lobe resection and a metastatic node. I'm not sure what she actually had the thoracotomy for.
3) Cardiorespiratory – COPD plus TR plus CABG with bioprosthetic AVR (no pHTN or RV failure). This was weird. Stem was: 'Mild SOB, please examine cardiorespiratory system'. I got confused and wasn't sure if they wanted a full cardiovascular exam and a full respiratory exam, ended up doing a 'half-arsed' mixed one (mostly cardio) because I thought I'd run out of time and ended up finishing too early instead. He had some signs of COPD with barrel chest and prolonged expiratory phase. Also had severe TR with raised JVP and pulsatile liver and a prominent (but not mechanical) second heart sound. So tried to tie it together as COPD with RV failure and pulmonary hypertension and severe functional TR.

And you had to pick up that he had had a CABG with vein harvest sites. The examiners said 'If I told you he has had a valve replacement, what do you think it would be?' and 'If I told you he had no functional impairment from his SOB, what do you think is the cause of his heart murmur?'. I had no idea what they wanted me to say. I thought 'flow murmur over a bioprosthetic AVR?' but then I wasn't sure why SOB was part of the stem … then the bell rang! Difficult case.

4) Rheumatology – CREST. Stem was: 'Examine the hands and proceed'. It was quite straightforward but I still freaked out anyway (rheumatology exam scares me and even the examiners commented on the fact I looked scared!). She had everything except calcinosis. She had clear lungs and no pulmonary hypertension. Then they showed me a hand X-ray and blood tests with positive anticentromere antibodies.

Paeds Point
Just like for long cases, our paediatric contributors felt the pool of paediatric short cases is just too small to write down.

27

Putting It All Together for the Clinical Exam – One Month Out

The content of what you say is very important in the Clinical Exam. By now, you have spent hours doing long and short cases, memorising diagnostic criteria, and can recite whole paragraphs of Talley and O'Connor.

In the month before the Clinical Exam, it is time to perfect your presentation style. It's about leaving the examiners thinking 'What a nice young doctor – reminds me of myself in some ways' or some such rosy sentiment. You don't want them to look at each other thinking 'Thank goodness he's not looking after my patients'.

What is Your Presentation Style?

Your presentation style is a vague phrase that encompasses all those subconscious things that affect what the examiners think about you, regardless of what you say. It includes what you look like, what your voice sounds like and how you phrase things. So much of communication is non-verbal. Cast your mind back to all those 'Body Language' TV shows in the 1980s. Remember how someone telling a lie always looks down and to the right? A nervous person shuffles their feet and folds their arms in front of them?

On Exam Day, most of us were nervous. If you practise being confident and calm before, it really does help on the day. It is also important to be true to yourself – we all revert to type on Exam Day!

How to Pass the RACP Written and Clinical Exams: The Insider's Guide,
Second Edition. Zoë Raos and Cheryl Johnson.
© 2017 John Wiley & Sons Ltd. Published 2017 by John Wiley & Sons Ltd.

General Advice About Style

- Walk in and shake the hand of both examiners firmly. Introduce yourself in a strong and clear voice. Practise this even if you feel like a chump.
- Stand with your hands neatly behind your back, or at the front. Many of us are natural 'hand talkers' but this is not the time to be using your hands. In the exam, flailing your hands around makes you look even more nervous – hold them tight!
- Look the examiner in the eye. If you can't manage that, look at them in between the eyebrows or the nose. Looking at the floor, the wall, your shoes or back at the patient makes you appear terrified (which you are, but don't make it worse for yourself!) or, worse still, uninterested and bored!
- Pause before you answer a question. If you are not sure what's required, ask for clarification. Better than going off on a tangent.
- Speak clearly and enunciate your words. Ask your study pals and consultants for feedback about how easy your speech is to understand. Try recording yourself to find out how often you say 'umm' and 'ahhh'. Then practise your 'new' speaking style every time you do a practice case so that it becomes natural to speak in a slow and articulate way.
- Use pauses in your long case. They break up the monologue and make it easier to listen to. For example, 'In summary...' and then a pause was quite a good clue to the examiners to wake up and listen because the problem list was coming.
- On the day, there will be two examiners and they take turns at being the lead. Direct your responses to the person who asked the question. There may also be an observer in the room, but don't be put off by them.
- Treat each case as a separate exam. The examiner doesn't know that you completely screwed up your last short case so try not to let it affect your performance for the rest of the day's cases. One short case is totally failable.
- Be enthusiastic! Not a total nut bar, but feign for the subject. Don't crush the examiner's spirit by implying that his whole specialty bores you senseless.
- Don't hurt the patient! EVER!

Personalities That Fail the Clinical Exam

Take a look at the examples below and think about whether you would pass these 'personalities' if you were an examiner. Now think about whether you recognise aspects of yourself in any of these types. If you do (be honest, there's a little bit of Cowboy in all of us), then train yourself out if it before the exam. Seek advice from seniors to lose those bad habits. Aim to be a professional, courteous, interested, calm, wise, intelligent and sensible junior consultant.

The Possum in the Headlights

Candidate visibly shaking as she enters the room, attempts to shake hands with examiners but ends up dropping briefcase and contents go everywhere. Examiner gives introductory stem. Candidate turns deathly white and appears to have turned to stone. Examiner eventually prods candidate to 'do something' and she moves hesitantly towards the patient. Patient assures her he doesn't bite but she looks unconvinced. Completes the examination (not the cardiovascular as asked but a very nice neuro exam nonetheless). Examiner asks for her findings and she again turns to stone. Eventually manages to ask in a quavering voice: 'Is it mitral valve prolapse?'.

Score
Examiners sigh with relief that the 15 minutes are up. Can't help but think that the candidate would probably have a heart attack herself if faced with a patient with one. Reassure each other that 'another year of experience' will help this candidate enormously.

Mr Slooow

Can be recognised by his ability to perform an examination at the pace of a glacier melting. Consequently, he can only really comment on the first two cranial nerves which seldom reveal the diagnosis. Examiners are overcome by an overwhelming urge to light a stick of dynamite under the candidate.

Score
Impossible to pass this candidate as he didn't finish!

The Cocky Bastard

Candidate swaggers into the room for a short case and gives an overly vigorous handshake. Barely waits until the end of the stem before launching into an enthusiastic and thorough examination. Proceeds to look at the fundi, nailfolds and plantar responses – masterfully done but somewhat unorthodox parts of a respiratory exam. After five minutes, turns to the examiners and says in a condescending tone, 'Well, this is clearly a textbook case of interstitial lung disease, need I go on?'. It's not, so the examiners try to gently redirect him. Alas, he will not be swayed from his diagnosis. Ends up listing all the reasons why this couldn't possibly be anything except interstitial lung disease, and implies that anyone who can't hear the crackles is not a real doctor. Looks at the X-ray and says it's uninterpretable because it's of such poor quality but definitely supports the diagnosis of ILD anyway.

Score

Examiners seethe at the little whipper-snapper who dared to disagree with them. Take great delight in failing him.

Can't See the Wood for the Trees

Candidate starts the long case quite well by correctly reporting that the patient had leukaemia when she was eight years old. Candidate then launches into an exceedingly thorough history of this leukaemia, including a list of every transfusion the patient ever received. Fifteen minutes later and the candidate is still listing off what outpatients appointments the patient went to in 1985.

   Eventually the examiners interrupt to ask what she thought of the patient's emphysema. Candidate looks puzzled; she obviously didn't ask the patient about this topic. Quickly recovers and starts on her 'COPD speech', including quoting the recent journal articles she has read about DNA subtype analysis. Mentions that a lung transplant would be a good idea. At this, both examiners' eyebrows shoot up. 'Really? Would you *really* attempt a transplant in a patient who is still smoking and lives in a car?'

Score

Candidate obviously knows a lot about medicine (in theory); she just doesn't seem to be able to connect it with the patient in front of her. Examiners happily fail the candidate, assuring each other that a dose of 'good ol' common sense' wouldn't go amiss.

The Rambler

You will know him by his hunched over posture while he mumbles the history to himself. The examiners will try and catch his eye to tell him to speak up but the Rambler never looks up. His history will continue to meander along in no particular order until the examiners are lulled into a dreamless sleep by his monotonous tone.

Score

Even the friendliest of examiners will struggle to pass someone who can't speak coherently.

The Newbie

Candidate skips into the room looking bright-eyed and bushy-tailed. Listens to the stem and then turns to open his bag. Appears dazzled by its contents; it's as if he has never seen such objects before. Tentatively picks up a tendon hammer and then puts it back in the bag. Eventually picks up a stethoscope and starts listening to the patient's chest. Keeps listening for five minutes until told to stop and move on. Candidate stands chewing on his lip, contemplating what to do next. Suddenly leaps into action as if struck by a brainwave – percussion! Completes a very thorough percussion display and then returns to his position of standing meditatively, waiting for inspiration to strike. Examiners put him out of his misery and start the questioning. Candidate says he thinks it might be mitral regurgitation but he's never seen a case before so is not quite sure. Asked if he would like to see an ECG, he replies, 'Ooh yes, what a good idea'.

Score

Examiners check candidate's name and number. Wonder if he is, in fact, a doctor at all, since the whole experience seemed like a complete novelty to him. Quickly decide on a 'fail' and hope that the candidate will know how to use his equipment next year.

The Parrot

Candidate sits down for the long case discussion and tries to quote the patient as accurately as possible. Examiners have strange feeling of déjà-vu – this sounds exactly like when they talked to the patient directly! The candidate continues to tell the examiners in great detail every symptom that the patient reported without making any attempt to attach any diagnoses to these symptoms. Despite the 70 pack/year smoking history, slowly progressive breathlessness and quiet breath sounds, she lists 'asthma' on the problem list; after all, that's what the patient said he had!

Score

The examiners look at each other with puzzled expressions. It was a perfect imitation of a patient giving a history but what they really wanted was a doctor interpreting a patient's symptoms and signs. Maybe another year of experience will teach her to act like a doctor and not merely report what the patient thinks is wrong.

The Cowboy

Candidate slopes into the room and attempts to high five the lead examiner. The examiner does not respond. Starts the long case discussion and seems to have discovered the main points. Seems a bit sketchy on some of the details and fails to mention anything about the home situation or family history. Starts presenting the examination findings by saying, 'I reckon the JVP was a little on the high side which means the patient could be a bit wet. The ankles were sort of puffy too, maybe heart failure; could be liver though'. The examiners ask if he examined the patient's gait, but it seems he did not. In fact, it seems like he missed out the whole neuro exam. Examiners give him some blood results to which he replies, 'Yeah, nah, looks OK to me'.

Score

Examiners thank their lucky stars the candidate doesn't work at their hospital since he seems so relaxed, a lawsuit must surely be just around the corner. Figure that a 'fail' might make him take this medicine gig a bit more seriously.

The Liar

Talk to any examiner and ask them their thoughts on candidates who 'make up' what the fundi looked like or try to bluff their way through a social history they haven't taken. Liars are the absolute worst of all.

Score

Instant fail. You have been warned.

The Whiner

Candidate starts his long case by complaining loudly that the patient seemed to have no idea what was wrong with him. Goes on to give the examiners a blow-by-blow description about how crappy the patient was and how it was probably a deliberate attempt by the patient to be 'difficult'. Eventually the examiners convince the candidate to present something, but he keeps returning to how his exam was sabotaged by the dumb patient. Ends by saying that he's not surprised the patient has no family support because he didn't seem like a very nice person and anyway, if people aren't going to help themselves …

Score

Examiner thinks of his own sweet mother with dementia and shudders at the thought that this candidate could be looking after her and blaming her for her own disease. Fails the candidate, hoping that he will develop some compassion and insight by next year. The worst thing is that the Whiner often feels incredibly hard done by because he got a long case patient with memory problems. He spends the next year feeling bitter and twisted (and often forgets to practise his approach to the confused or difficult patient).

Summary

Your presentation style needs to be confident, humble, yet true to who you are as an individual for both long and short cases.

Some of the above personalities might seem a bit extreme (you'd be surprised, though!) but the concepts still stand. Candidates don't fail because they don't know their stuff – they fail because they *come across* as if they don't know their stuff.

So remember:

- control your anxiety by practising under exam conditions
- practise doing your cases in the time allotted
- be humble and respectful of your patients and seniors
- never *ever* make up signs or symptoms even if they 'should' be there
- think about the big picture and be more holistic than you have ever been before
- practise using your equipment and make sure you can do tricky things like nailfolds
- interpret the symptoms and signs you are given, don't just list what the patient told you
- list only the relevant differentials for this patient (how likely is kala azar really?)
- be formal and don't use slang or abbreviations no matter how widely they are used in everyday practice or in this book (that includes JVP!)
- don't whinge – you can mention it once and then drop it.

28

The Lead-Up to the Exam

The Week Before

You've practised hard for weeks, you've had a relaxing few days leading up to the exam to settle your nerves and you've been repeating the phrase 'I deserve to pass' like some sort of mantra. This is how to make sure that all your hard work culminates in a great performance on the day.

The final week before the exam is tiger country. Everything in your very being tells you that a few more long cases and a few shorts just might make all the difference. Resist the impulse! Past candidates have done this and been slain in a practice long case mere days before the exam (now why would any consultant think this was helpful?). Consequently, the candidate is a quivering mess of insecurity and self-doubt on the day of the exam. In effect, that one final long case undid months of good work and preparation in one fell swoop.

If you listen to nothing else we say in this book, for Pete's sake, don't do ANY long or short cases in the final week!

You will need something to occupy your time in that final week (between relaxing massages and positive visualisation). We recommend you take out all your old long cases and re-read them. You may be able to work out ways of structuring them slightly differently now that you see them again. You could also go through a few key favourite short cases and check that you can recite the signs of severity in aortic stenosis. But be careful. The final week is about backing off so that on the day, you will see the big picture and won't be distracted by the details. Journal articles, new diseases to learn about and new approaches in your technique are all totally banned.

How to Pass the RACP Written and Clinical Exams: The Insider's Guide, Second Edition. Zoë Raos and Cheryl Johnson.
© 2017 John Wiley & Sons Ltd. Published 2017 by John Wiley & Sons Ltd.

Just like in the Written Exam, make sure any travel arrangements are set in stone and allow for delays. If you need any convincing, just ask the candidates who were caught in a snowstorm at the top of the South Island that closed the airport. They drove for hours through the night in a taxi to the exam centre. Many of them failed. The College does not make allowances for candidates who have issues with travel.

Be cunning. What type of patient is likely to be at your exam centre? Who is organising the exam and what is their specialty? Is this a transplant centre? Is there a big oncology service? Is a geriatrician organising the exam? Is it a small regional hospital? Is there a particular demographic served by that hospital? If you are lucky and know who the organiser is, then you will know he or she will collect their own patients for the day more than any other type of patient (this means that you are stuffed if the organiser is a general physician or paediatrician – anything goes).

Check out Chapter 33 for more information on how the clinical exam is organised and the day is run.

The Day Before

Odds are your exam centre is in a hospital where you've never worked and in a city where you've never been. Arrive the day before, work out how to get to the exam centre, where to park (if you're driving) and where the exam is located. You don't want to be running around madly looking for Building 53 with five minutes to spare.

The Morning of the Exam – Staying Calm

Try and get someone to drive you to the exam, either a taxi driver or loved one. Our nerves were shot and we might have caused an accident if we'd tried to negotiate a motorway that day.

Get there early and be prepared for delays with traffic, fog, rain and floods. Take into account time spent looking for a carpark (can you tell we come from Auckland?). Arriving anything more than 10 minutes early at the actual exam centre is very irritating to the exam organisers. By all means, get to the hospital early, work out where you are going and when, and then chill out on a park bench or in the cafeteria until shortly before the reporting time. There is nothing more irritating than the super-eager candidate as the organisers are trying to direct patients into their rooms and corral the examiners. Our advice in Chapter 9 about looking after yourself before the Written Exam and avoiding stress cadets is just as important now.

Consider arranging someone to meet you for lunch or eat your lunch alone or with trusted study buddies. Avoid the stress cadets who will be dissecting each case from the morning in minute detail. Escape for a break or bring a novel or some music – depending on how your day is scheduled, it can be a long lunch break.

Getting Through Exam Day – Tips From Registrars

- Make **eye contact** with the examiners – it forces you to look up and project your voice rather than mumbling into your notes.
- Ask for the **medication list** as soon as you introduce yourself in the long case. It's a good pointer to problems the patient may not remember to tell you. (Yes, patients have been known to 'forget' about their kidney transplant!) Ask the patient these three questions in the long case:
  - 'What did the examiners talk to you about?'
  - 'What did the examiners examine?'
  - 'Have we discussed anything that the examiners did not discuss?'

  And if you are struggling with the case, ask these questions more than once! I got crucial information when I felt like I was missing something and asked the questions again.
- Don't expect the day to go exactly as you expect or expect it to be like what's described in the books. You don't necessarily get to present a lot.
- They will try to gently nudge you off target and **out of your comfort zone** so be prepared to adjust quickly. **It's OK to pause for a while** (even for half a minute) while you gather your thoughts – lots of very good orators do this. Churchill, for example, deliberately scripted pauses into his speeches for maximum effect. The delivery adds power to the message. It's also OK to ask for clarification of a question.

- **Keep talking!** Even if you think you are failing miserably, you might not be. Silence is *not* golden in the long case discussion.
- Best advice is to **get a good rapport** with the patient if you can. My patients seemed to have been told that they shouldn't just give the information to me and I should have to extract it from them. You have to have good rapport with them to get the good stuff!
- Try and **finish the long case history and examination within 40–45 minutes**, allowing you time to prepare and think. The examiners will ask you questions you don't know the answer to (hopefully, they won't be things like 'what was the patient's name?'). **If you don't know the answer, *say so*** and say that you would consult a colleague or book for the information. This is what you would do in real life and proves that you have a safe way of practising. Don't guess what you would do – it implies to the consultants that you might also guess drug doses too.
- The weirdest thing on the day was the **complete absence of feedback**. The examiners are trained to be poker-faced. They give nothing away about your performance. So much so that I wanted to go home at lunchtime and cry into a good Irish stout. But I went back for the afternoon and passed somehow.
- On the day, there will be two examiners. They seem to take turns at being the lead. **Direct your responses to the person who asked the question**.
- **Treat each case as a separate exam.** The examiner doesn't know that you completely screwed up your last short case so try not to let it affect your performance for the rest of the day's cases. One short case is totally failable.
- **Expect to recognise an examiner or two.** If you come from a big centre, you may well have 2–3 examiners who you know or may have even worked with. Try not to think of them as 'nephrologists' since they are meant to 'general physicians' for the sake of the exam.

Final Advice From Examiners

It's always interesting to hear the examiners' side of the story. Over the years, they have seen hundreds of registrars sit this exam and have a pretty good idea of what works and what doesn't. Some of this advice is repeated. If so, it's because it's a very important point to make.

- We know you know all of the facts (after all, you passed the Written Exam which is more than your examiners are currently capable of). Instead, we want to know about the **art of medicine as well as the science**.
- Do not do the exam if you (or someone who knows you well, e.g. a supervisor) do not believe you should be there. **Your lack of self-belief comes across** when you are presenting yourself. Give yourself another year and work hard on your self-belief.
- **Do not cram**; this is not a test of knowledge but of clinical ability. You will acquire this through clinical work and structured mock cases.
- **Engage the examiners in discussion**. Try and keep control of things rather than letting the examiner be in absolute control. Be interested in what you are saying rather than being a robot reading a piece of paper.
- **Say 'I don't know' if you don't**. If you are uncertain, then say that you are but say what you think might be right answer. You can always be corrected.
- **Avoid people who are 'high pressure' pre-exam**. This will upset entirely adequate preparation and make you question whether you really are good enough to pass (just because you haven't done 70 practice long cases). Everyone is different so try not to compare yourself with others.
- When practising the cases, **do not be nice to each other**. If you are hard on each other for missing things, it raises the bar and then the actual exam is much less scary, making passing the exam easier.
- **Be well presented** with nothing that will distract the examiners; dramatic fashion statements, messy or casual clothing, dirty hair, extravagant jewellery and excessively strong perfume might all divert the examiner away from concentrating on your knowledge.
- **Never, never, NEVER tell a fib**. If you haven't done something, admit it. We all forget things and we all know the effects of the pressure of the exam. If you have omitted something, say so rather than getting caught out.
- **Present the positives and pertinent negatives**. Avoid presenting a large amount of irrelevant data.
- **Make sure you are competent** in all aspects of the physical exam. After all these years of training, you should be competent in the basics!
- There is no point in examining where there is no gain simply to demonstrate a technique, e.g. vocal fremitus.

- **Listen carefully to the examiners**. If they ask you the same question in several different ways, you are likely to be on the wrong track and they are throwing you a life-line.
- If the questions seem to be getting progressively harder, **don't automatically panic**. The examiners are trying to plumb the depth of your knowledge and an exceptional candidate might be pushed very hard. If someone is failing, the examiners don't need to ask hard questions. That is why those who get distinction often think they have done badly, while those who fail seem to think there were no hard questions and can't see where they went wrong.
- **Do not make things up**. Every single examiner who contributed to this book kept saying this again and again and AGAIN! Maybe they are trying to tell us something.
- If you see an examiner after the exam, **don't try and find out how well you did**. It might be embarrassing for all concerned.
- **Don't arrive too early**. Whilst it is understandable to arrive early and be prepared, it is difficult to separate candidates and patients who arrive at the same time. By all means, arrive at the venue early for a coffee but arrive at the actual examination area close to your reporting time. It does not help anyone to see a patient prior to walking into the examination room.
- **Try not to 'lose it' if you have a bad case**. It happens to the best of candidates. It is vitally important to move on so that it does not affect the rest of your exam. Once the doors close on the case, close your mind and forget about it. Focus on the next one.

Summary

- DO NOT DO ANY CASES IN THE WEEK OF THE EXAM! NONE!
- In the week of the exam, go over your previous long cases, review common short cases and RELAX!
- Scope out the exam venue the day before but do not arrive too early on the day.
- Do not lie or make up signs. It is better to say you don't know or that you forgot to check for a particular sign.
- Once the door closes on a 'bad' case, forget about it and move on … don't let it affect the rest of your day.

Section 3

The F-words – Freedom, Failure, Feedback, Family, Finding Patients and Fellowship

29

The Post-Exam World

Wow! I Passed!

What do registrars say it is like to pass?

- 'Weird, especially if you expected to fail. I went home and had a nap then felt a lot better.'
- 'Slightly anticlimactic. I felt really deflated and at a loss as to what to do. And then I felt guilty for not feeling happier.'
- 'I kept checking my candidate number on the website, not believing I could have passed. But I did! It was like winning the lotto. My boss gave me the afternoon off. I felt really bad for my colleagues who didn't pass, they worked so hard.'
- 'A relief! We found out at work and it was like a party – finding out about my friends and congratulating everybody. I don't think I did much work that day!'

From all of us at How To Pass, well done. We are very proud. You survived the Written Exam and nailed the Clinical. Your future is looking bright and options are opening up. Take a moment to enjoy your hard-won success. Then, if you are a Kiwi, you are in for a rather rude shock as in about 72 hours, you will have to decide what advanced training programme to apply for and get ready for interviews. Don't panic … turn to Chapters 34 and 35.

How to Pass the RACP Written and Clinical Exams: The Insider's Guide,
Second Edition. Zoë Raos and Cheryl Johnson.
© 2017 John Wiley & Sons Ltd. Published 2017 by John Wiley & Sons Ltd.

Oh. I've Failed

Failing the Clinical Exam is really tough. If this book could take you through to its office, get you a cup of tea, sit you down, smile and frown at the right moments as you go through blow by blow what went well and what was awful ... it would. Instead, please to turn to Chapter 30, which will hopefully help you feel a bit better and (when you're ready) describe how to maximise your chances of passing next year.

The Official Feedback Session

In our day, you passed the Clinical Exam or you didn't. If you passed, that was the end of the correspondence from the College (unless you won the medal). If you failed, you got detailed feedback in a meeting with a local examiner or the Director of Physician Education. Now, everyone (successful or not) gets individualised written feedback from each case, copied directly from the examiners' notes on the day. How valuable!

For unsuccessful candidates, you can use this information in your feedback meeting with your DPE (or other named consultant) as this will help you prepare for your next attempt. One such candidate thought the feedback session made her feel better about how she had performed. She thought she had totally mucked up one long case and was surprised to find that she had passed it. The examiner gave her some useful advice on how to improve. Make the most of your feedback session by asking questions and clarifying areas you need to work on.

For successful candidates, you will get a great idea of your own performance and get a bit of marking moderation so you will be in hot demand for practice long cases next year. For those who have not yet sat, if you are so fortunate, ask some recent sitters if they would share their feedback forms with you and ask them about the cases they had and how it went on the day.

Summary

- Passing is awesome! Congratulations! Enjoy your hard-earned success. We are very proud.
- Failing is the pits. You are not alone. Please go to Chapter 30 for support and guidance.

30

How to Fail – The Outsider's Guide to the FRACP Exam

Introduction

One of the nicest things about writing a book about passing exams is hearing from candidates who have triumphed, and that this little book was a help. This genuinely warms the cockles of the heart – what a satisfying feeling to have contributed in a small way to another's success.

The warm fuzzies scampered when Roderick Ryan emailed to say the book needed work, not just to help people pass but to offer more support to candidates who fail. And how they can rise above the pain to pass. Rod was kind enough to contribute.

Chapter Author: Dr Roderick Ryan, General Physician, Box Hill Hospital and Maroondah Hospital, Victoria

I have more experience in failing the Written and Clinical Exams than anyone has in passing them. I have organised clinical teaching at my hospital since 2004 and am an experienced local examiner for the Clinical Exam. After a particular candidate passed their first Clinical after their third attempt at the Written Exam, I decided that not enough was written about what to do if you fail. This chapter is based on my own experiences, and those of people I know who have all been in the unenviable position of failure.

How to Pass the RACP Written and Clinical Exams: The Insider's Guide, Second Edition. Zoë Raos and Cheryl Johnson.
© 2017 John Wiley & Sons Ltd. Published 2017 by John Wiley & Sons Ltd.

'I Failed the FRACP Exam – What Shall I Do?'

Maintain Self-Belief in the Face of Failure

It can be hard to maintain self-belief in the face of failing the Written or Clinical. For many candidates, these may be the first exams they have ever failed after many years of stellar achievement at school and university. This is a lonely time, especially while your friends are celebrating. Always remember that you are doing a high-level job and you are doing it well. You have failed this exam and while that feels awful, you surely have not failed at every aspect of your life, such as being a registrar, being a partner or being a friend. Try and maintain perspective. You are not the first person to fail this exam and will not be the last. You can therefore progress to passing like countless thousands before you.

Take Personal Responsibility for Failure

Don't blame those close to you, be they friends, colleagues, parents, siblings, partner or children. The exam is your responsibility. They share the stress of you doing it, but they should not bear the burden of you failing it.

Think About a Location Change – Hospital, City or Job

Sometimes change, be it deliberate or forced upon you, can be a good thing. You get a fresh start, a new perspective, new people who can help you, and potentially an added bonus that you avoid running into your former residents (or students!) who have passed the exam before you do. Change can be as small as changing the type of job you are doing (for instance, leaving ICU fellow jobs behind and going back to general medicine), changing hospitals within a city, moving to another city/state or making a big move across the Tasman.

The Two Lists of People Who Can Help You Pass

I liked to imagine two lists of people in my head – one list was people who had supported me through my training and who I wanted to pass for, to repay their faith. The other list (mercifully small) was the people who had no faith in me, for whom I wanted to pass to prove that they were wrong. Over time, the first list mattered much more, and what's more, I realised that some on my second list really should have been on the first list, but I was too blind to see it.

Visualise Your Future

As I left each hospital after the exam, I said to myself that I would return when I received my FRACP and get a photo of myself outside that hospital with my diploma. I have subsequently taken some of these photos, starting with the hospital where I passed – also lining up all my family for a photo (they suffered through it all as much as I did).

Once You Pass, Help Others, Especially 'Repeaters'

When you pass the exam, I think you should help others pass. If you have experienced failure, you are ideally positioned to help others in a similar situation.

Tips for Coping with Failure in the Written Exam

Within a couple of weeks of receiving the news that your attempt was unsuccessful, you will get an A4 sheet including a breakdown of all your marks, and which topics you passed and didn't pass. All candidates get this feedback. It is quite comprehensive and compares your individual performance with the average score of all the candidates in each subspecialty and overall. According to the College website, candidates can request a re-mark of the MCQ papers.

For future study, focus on areas of weakness where you did poorly in the exam. Make a particular effort to read about and understand the principles underlying that area, going right back to the basics (physiology, pharmacology, anatomy and biochemistry) if necessary.

Take a break from study to regroup before re-embarking on preparation for the Written Exam. Do things you used to do such as read, play sport and go out. Set a deadline for recommencing study again – for most resitters anywhere from three to six months is adequate.

Schedule productive study sessions. Try not to study when tired – this is very important, though obviously very difficult for most medical and paediatric registrars. If you have a noisy or distracting household, study at the hospital, university or local library to work in a quiet environment without interruptions. Two hours at the local library is more productive than eight hours with small children and the dog howling outside the door. The small children will howl less when you arrive back from the library, with more time to spend with them.

Get fit. It may sound strange but as a doctor, your fitness levels have probably fallen, especially while studying for the exam. You learn better when you are fitter. You will sleep better too. There are robust studies demonstrating that memory is more effective after physical exercise.

Be organised and plan your year. Join a productive study group. Secure your place on a two-week exam preparation course (ideally a different course from the previous year). Plan your study and annual leave carefully.

Many candidates who fail reflect that they did not focus enough on old exam questions nor learn to think in an MCQ way. They thought knowing the basics was enough, and didn't spend enough time on the questions. If this is true for you, then focus your revision heavily on MCQ-style studying. When you practise an old question, go beyond the question. Why is the examiner asking this question? What point is s/he trying to make? Which two responses can clearly be chucked? Do I really know enough about this topic, or do I need to brush up on the basics to really understand it? In addition to FRACP questions, MKSAPs and the MRCP question bank are a better way to get your brain in MCQ mode and uncover deficits in knowledge than aimlessly reading articles, lecture notes and textbooks.

Tips for Coping with Failure in the Clinical Exam

After – Accept That You Failed, Even If 'Unlucky'

Failing the Written Exam is tough. Some find failing the Clinical tougher, and somehow more personal. It is important to accept that you failed, as this acceptance helps you cycle through the Kübler-Ross stages of grief quickly. Even if you feel unlucky or 'hard done by', as I did having once passed both long cases and two of the four short cases. A fail is a fail, and a close fail shows you that you are getting on the right track.

Self-Reflection – Write Down Why You Failed

Before getting the feedback from your DPT, write down why you think you failed. Then compare this to the feedback from your supervisor. It has been shown that among people who lose their jobs or fail to get jobs from an interview, those who write about why this happened and what they are going to do about it are more likely to quickly find new jobs.

Speaking Clubs (Rostrum, Toastmasters) or Acting Lessons

Your medical career does not really train you to be a public speaker or to be confident asserting your opinion in front of strangers and people in authority. It can be worthwhile joining a speaking club – there are many such clubs throughout Australia and New Zealand, such as Rostrum and Toastmasters. Some candidates have even joined acting classes to improve their confidence and presentation skills.

Seven Key Clinical Exam Skills that Must be Mastered by Those Who Have Failed

1   Nail your Short Case Routines

Practise your examination technique on normal subjects for all the major short cases – cardiology, respiratory, cranial nerves, neurological upper and lower limbs, abdomen, rheumatological and gait examinations. These need to be rote learned on normal subjects until they can be done in your sleep. Normal subjects can be your family, flatmates, study group members or patients on the ward.

Once you have the short case examinations on a normal subject down pat, use your imagination and add in some practice pathology. For example, pretend your flatmate has severe aortic stenosis, parkinsonian gait, rheumatoid hands or a lower motor neurone disease and practise presenting these findings.

Take medical students for short cases, with you as examiner. Not only will you become a very popular registrar, it is extremely helpful to see cases from the other side. It becomes very clear what you, the examiner, like to see in candidates. Also, practise being the examiner for other trainees. Putting yourself in the role of examiner gets you used to knowing what examiners are likely to ask about, and the sorts of responses that annoy them.

Practising short cases on real patients is obviously very important, but make sure that you have the routines absolutely down pat first.

2   Perfect Your Short Case Summaries

You will be marked on your examination technique, finding signs as well as for presenting your findings in an orderly way. Practise your summaries. Using video to look at your 'performance' is an excellent way to iron out bad habits.

Make the most of short case practice sessions at the hospital. Once you have finished your case, including the presentation, question time and feedback session, ask the examiner to help you 'redo' the summary statement of findings and differential diagnosis to a gold standard. You can then practise this gold standard summary in the mirror when you get home. File this away for future study.

3   Do Enough Long Cases Over the Whole Year

Make sure you do enough long cases. You will have 10 months of preparation time, which puts you at a real advantage. Consider doing one long case under exam conditions every 2–4 weeks while the next lot of candidates are studying for their Written Exam. Do long cases with senior registrars and consultants who are tough but fair, who will give accurate feedback but also honest advice about improving your performance.

4   Improving Your Long Case Presentation

As per the short cases, 'redo' the summary statement and problem list after getting feedback to the gold standard. Re-present the same case to a different examiner, to practise how it could have been done better. File the record of each long case for reading over at a later time. Video some of your presentations so you can analyse your performance and improve it.

5   Get Your Long Case Timing Right

Timing is a big reason why candidates fail their long case. If you spend the next four months getting the timing right for your long cases, you have done well.

6   See a Wide Variety of Patients

As the months go by, you will notice gaps in the types of patients you have seen. Use the extra months to fill in these gaps. For example, plan ahead, take a day off and travel to a tertiary transplant centre and arrange two or three practice long cases. Look for other gaps in your experience and knowledge. You could spend an afternoon in a rheumatology or gastroenterology clinic as an extra person. Call or email well ahead – senior trainees and fellows are happy to supervise cases in their area of specialty even if you have never met them before, especially when you are not competing with dozens of other candidates.

7   Handling Question Time – Practise Being an Examiner

Join up with other trainees who are resitting their Clinical Exam and ask to be 'second examiner' when colleagues present their long cases and vice versa. Offer to be an examiner for medical student long case sessions. This makes you think about what examiners will ask about, and thus gets you prepared for the lines of questioning when you present. This role reversal is crucial for candidates who have failed. Hopefully, you will no longer see the examiners as enemies, as you have walked in their shoes a few times and can understand their point of view.

Snakes and Ladders

In the past, the FRACP Exams were a game of Snakes and Ladders. Candidates would battle through multiple attempts at the Written Exam, finally pass, fail five attempts at the Clinical Exam then could re-sit the Written Exam again. Candidates could spend years and years rolling the dice, moving along the squares, sliding down snakes and hauling themselves up ladders. Failing the Written Exam after doing Clinical Exams was like that really big snake on the Snakes and Ladders board that takes you from near the end to almost back to the start. In my training, I slid down that massive snake prompting a huge degree of self-examination. In the end, despite everything, I decided to go around the board again. I appreciated a 'quiet' winter and enjoyed other parts of my life that year. I finally passed.

Times have changed for the RACP. No more Snakes and Ladders. As of 2017, trainees are allowed three attempts at the Written Exam. If you fail that last attempt, then you can no longer train. The same is true for the Clinical Exam. Three attempts – that's it. There are time limits on completing basic and advanced training and changing requirements. There are transition plans for candidates who have already attempted exams pre-2017. Check the college website for more information. The RACP has put considerable effort to support trainees in difficulty. If you're having problems passing Exams, get help. Your local DPE will support you. We suggest you enlist battle-weary consultants who have been in your shoes too.

Summary

- You are not alone. Many have failed the Written and/or Clinical Exams, gone on to pass and are now well established physicians and paediatricians.
- You can always get better. Everyone can improve their knowledge and MCQ skills for the Written Exam.
- Timing and presentation skills for the Clinical are crucial. Use the extra months to your advantage.
- It is worthwhile to put yourself in the examiners' position in Clinical Exam practice.
- A year to wait to resit an exam seems like a long time. I often compare it to Olympians like Hicham El Guerrouj, the dominant male 1500 metres runner and World Record holder for many years. Despite being the heavy favourite at the 2000 Sydney Olympics, he came second and, like all Olympic athletes, he had to wait *four years* for redemption, which came at the 2004 Athens Olympics.

31

Paying It Forward – How to Provide Feedback for Practice Cases

We have given and received great, average and terrible feedback over the years. We wouldn't have passed our exam without kind consultants who took time out of their schedules to whip us into shape. Now we are out the other side, a plethora of workshops, websites and higher degrees are dedicated to feedback. We have written this chapter not to replace a Master's thesis in medical education, but to give a rough guide from the frontline so feedback for Clinical Exam practice can be a time-efficient, constructive and useful educational experience for you, whether you're giving it (feedback- er) or getting it (feedback-ee). This includes supervising friends and peers pre-exam, and consultants and senior registrars providing feedback to junior colleagues.

The first aim is that the feedback-er gives the feedback-ee an accurate and honest picture of his or her performance. The performance is ideally measured against the expected standard. Next, the feedback-er's job is to communicate what about the performance was below, at or above that standard. Finally, the feedback-er needs to provide the feedback-ee with specific ways to improve their performance next time.

The literature makes much of encouraging candidates to assess their own performance. There is a place for this but it takes most candidates a fair few practice cases to be able to participate in useful self-appraisal. Close to exam time, you could ask the candidate 'How did that go for you?' at the start of the feedback session.

Just as the candidates have to get their tone and style right, it helps if feedback-ers do too. If you have to be very honest as the candidate stuffed up in biblical proportions, have a phrase up your sleeve like 'I know this is hard, but better to hear this from me today than on the

How to Pass the RACP Written and Clinical Exams: The Insider's Guide,
Second Edition. Zoë Raos and Cheryl Johnson.
© 2017 John Wiley & Sons Ltd. Published 2017 by John Wiley & Sons Ltd.

marking schedule from the College in a month's time.' Ripping to shreds is seldom useful. We know two candidates who were on track to pass, did long cases that didn't go well for practical reasons the week before and were derailed by overly harsh practice examiners. They failed their Clinical Exam that year. Also, no favours are done by saying 'That was great!' when it was below average and remedial action is needed, especially early on in the lead-up.

The Feedback Loop

Think of feedback as being a bit like an audit loop. Jumping straight to the fun bit at the end by throwing ideas around and seeing what works is better than nothing, but a proper process will be more satisfactory, and reinforce change and improvement in quality over time.

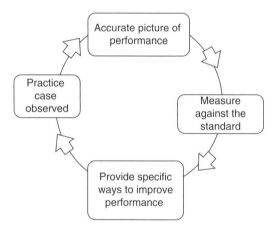

The Feedback Loop

Feedback for Clinical Exams

Once you've agreed to supervise a short or long case, we suggest turning to Chapter 12 and copying the marking schedule. This will give you the College's standard for passing, and also what to look for with candidates who are clearly struggling or excelling. Don't worry too much if you're a hard or easy marker, as the schedule will help – the important thing is to make the feedback-ee aware of the level they are aiming for, and how he or she measured up.

Once the feedback-er has given a fair and accurate appraisal of the feedback-ee and measured it against the expected standard, the fun begins – giving specific ways to improve performance. Try not to overwhelm with so many tips that the feedback-ee loses sight of what is important. Pick three or four main areas, and how to go about improving performance for next time. A bit of humour can go a long way, but can also backfire spectacularly with a sensitive candidate. This is a crazy and highly stressful time for our registrars – it's a balancing act between supporting them with empathy whilst being honest and whipping them into shape.

It is important that all feedback is constructive, positive or negative. Saying 'That was excellent' is not as useful as 'You'd get a 6/7 in the problem list and management sections, that integration with diabetes risk factors and the complex social situation was perfect'. Conversely, 'You failed that, you need to practise more' is not as useful as 'You're running out of time – if you don't finish you just can't pass your case. Your examination technique for the cranial nerves is okay. I suggest practising keeping to time on healthy volunteers for the next few days, then book in for another supervised cranial nerve short case'.

Some feedback-ers eschew this style, and don't give numerical marks. They prefer to give feedback on style, offering a range of detailed critiques from the case in a discussion with the candidate. This is still useful feedback. Candidates generally value any feedback at all, but always include whether you think the candidate passed or not as part of your discussion.

Below are more elements in long and short case presentations that are not necessarily included in the College marking schedule but are crucial for passing. Cast your mind back to your own exams, especially any Jedi mind tricks that helped you overcome nervousness, and pass this wisdom on.

Time

One of the most useful ways you can help a candidate is with his or her time management for both short and long cases.

Constructive Feedback Ideas

Use a stopwatch (there's one on your smartphone!) while observing the candidate. For a short case, note how long it took to finish the examination, how long the presentation took, and how long the grilling lasted. For the long case, note how long the candidate took to get to the problem list, and also discuss how time management went in the room with the patient.

Style

Style is the way in which a candidate presents himself or herself to an examiner. Nerves can mean that the most intelligent and friendly registrar can fumble, mumble and totally guff up. Have a read of Chapter 27 for personalities that fail the exam and see if you can spot one!

Short case examination style is well covered in the marking schedule in Chapter 23. Was the examination routine a slick, well-practised affair? Did the candidate help put the patient at ease? Was there fluency from demonstrating one sign to the next? Did they miss anything out? Did they complete the exam in the appropriate time? Did they spend too long on one particular aspect?

Constructive Feedback Ideas

This will depend on the area of difficulty. Many candidates need to practise their routine, keep to time and receive honest feedback about how their style appears to an examiner and tips on overcoming nerves.

Speech

Did the candidate talk too quickly or too slowly? Was he or she easy to understand or was there too much mumbling? Did the candidate pause and use verbal signposts? Was the long case presentation a tedious 15-minute monotone that sent you to sleep? Was your candidate overly excitable and resembled a Labrador puppy? How many fillers (um, ahhh, well, basically…) were used? Was the presentation fluent or did the candidate stumble from one point to the next?

Constructive Feedback Ideas

If the presentation was a verbal dog's breakfast, it can be constructive for the candidate to go home, write the whole thing out perfectly, record using the video function on a smartphone and play back. Some practice examiners tally verbal fillers as a teaching point to snap the candidate out of the habit. If the candidate is a 'basically' addict, try swapping for 'essentially' – it sounds a bit better. Teach about pausing for effect, and how to get tone right in the exam situation.

Eye Contact

Did the candidate spend the entire time talking to the floor, ceiling or notes? Did a large manila folder dwarf the candidate and get in the way of the presentation? Did they make adequate amounts of eye contact?

Constructive Feedback Ideas

Eye contact is a tricky one. It can be overdone and underdone and the acceptable amount varies between individuals. If you notice no eye contact with your candidate, suggest the old trick of looking at the examiner's nose.

Nervous Habits

Some candidates are flagrant hand talkers. Others act out the entire examination routine on themselves. Some have a nervous cough, jiggle their legs, pick their nails, sweat, talk incredibly quickly or bite their lips.

Constructive Feedback Ideas

It is easy (and very important) to identify a nervous habit because they distract examiners. It can be harder to give advice about remedying it. Usually a Jedi mind trick is needed. For example, one of the authors talks fast, uses her hands like a flamenco dancer and has the worst poker face. When nervous, she just about takes flight. For the exam, she had to hold her stethoscope in a death grip behind her back to stop her hands from distracting the examiners and imagine talking at half normal pace. This unnamed author also high-fived a patient at the end of an Exam short case. Not recommended. Resist the high-five.

Overall Look

This seems shallow, but it isn't. Getting that balance of looking smart yet appropriate is important (refer to Chapter 13). Doctors present themselves professionally to inspire confidence in themselves, their team and their patients. It is totally OK to be an individual, but if there is something annoying or distracting, feed this back. Can your candidate elicit a knee jerk without ripping a seam? For short cases, how does your candidate interact with their equipment – do they look puzzled every time the kit bag is opened or do you see confidence and efficiency?

Constructive Feedback Ideas

Be honest but kind.

- 'When you bend over, your undies show. Get a longer shirt.'
- 'My kids would love your Doc McStuffin briefcase; have you thought about a black one for the actual exam?'
- 'Fun bright pink lippy! On Exam Day, go for chapstick.'
- 'Has anyone mentioned to you about body odour? Better to hear this from me than to make the wrong impression on Exam Day. I'd suggest buying seven new cotton shirts, wash or dry clean after every wear and use antiperspirant and antibacterial soap every day too. It will really help your confidence on Exam Day, so get into the routine before then.'

Long Case History and Examination Findings

There is excellent stuff in the marking schedule on Chapter 15. Mention any glaring omissions. Did the candidate cover the examination findings well? What important negative or positive findings did they omit? Was it all presented in the right time frame? What aspect did the candidate spend too much time on?

Discuss different phrases that summarise key parts of the history and examination succinctly. Discuss how to emphasise important findings and minimise minutiae. Often this is a time management issue – candidates can spend three minutes on negative exam findings and not finish their problem list, so point this out and offer solutions.

Problem List

This is really important. Every candidate and feedback-er has a different technique for putting together a problem list (see Chapters 15 & 16) so this can make feedback tricky. It can be too easy to criticise and nit-pick, when in reality the candidate made a good fist of the problem list. There is room for subjectivity and individuality, but some candidates leave out very important problems or fail to emphasise key aspects. You can help. How well did they structure the problem list? Was it in order of relevance? Did the candidate add problems that are irrelevant (cardiovascular risk factor modification in a 20 year old with Crohn's) and miss something important (smoking cessation in a 20 year old with Crohn's)?

Did the candidate's problem list match up with your own? Discuss ways to prioritise, organise and refine the problem list. Give some advice on talking up the big stuff and how to 'mention and move on' through less important issues.

Discussion

This is tricky to mark, but so very important. The discussion hinges on the problem list. Again, the marking schedule will help. How well did they answer your questions or interpret investigations? Did they pause to think about the answer before it came out of their mouth? Did they answer the questions directly or did they meander their way to a strange conclusion? Did the candidate get flustered? A lot of candidates come unstuck in the discussion part because they 'revert to type' and can get too cocky, too dithery or too mumbly.

Constructive Feedback Ideas

Discuss ways of structuring responses, having 'down-pat' responses to common questions, how to answer questions directly, how to pause and think and how to work with the candidate's personality style to keep the examiners on side.

Summary

- Being a practice examiner takes time and effort. Thank you for doing it, we've never heard of anyone who has passed this exam without good souls like you stepping up to the plate.
- The feedback loop is a time-efficient way of giving feedback that works for the feedback-er and the feedback-ee.
- Some examiners don't like to give a formal mark and prefer detailed feedback. That's OK, but always include whether you think the candidate passed or failed. This is what candidates want and need to know.
- If the candidate failed the exam or underperformed, be honest and constructive. Discuss specific areas to work on to improve their performance next time.
- If the candidate did well, say so! By all means offer criticism, but it is important to emphasise the positives too.
- If your schedule allows, offer to review the candidate again to assess his or her progress. If you can't do this in person, it is still highly valuable for the candidate if you offer to read a perfected, 'typed up' case and offer further feedback.

32

Studying for the Exams with a Family on Board

Introduction

Cheryl and I had kids after we'd passed our exams. As we juggled two busy boys around book planning meetings, we'd ask each other 'How do they do it?' How do mums and dads fit in family life *and* work *and* study? And how can mums and dads have much less time, but often pass whereas those with fewer commitments freak out more and may not get through? We asked Rob, one of the registrars who passed his written and clinical first time, to write some wise words. Those of you without kids could learn a thing or two about time management from this chapter.

Chapter Author: Dr Robert Wakuluk, Advanced Trainee, Auckland

Since I got married and had kids, I have been much better at managing my time; it is much more precious. When I had seven hours of free time at med school, I would study effectively for two hours then waste the other five fretting and mucking around. For my FRACP exams, I hardly ever had more than two hours to myself, so had to study effectively for those two hours. It is important to stay involved with your family and try to find a healthy balance between work, studying and family life. If planned well, it is much healthier mentally and doesn't feel like the exam has too much of a detrimental effect. I noted that fellow candidates who were single or didn't have children spent all

How to Pass the RACP Written and Clinical Exams: The Insider's Guide,
Second Edition. Zoë Raos and Cheryl Johnson.
© 2017 John Wiley & Sons Ltd. Published 2017 by John Wiley & Sons Ltd.

their time studying but appeared much more stressed all the time. Having family can put things in perspective.

Preparing for the exams is far more complicated with a family, but it can be done. Some lucky people are able to study in the evening after getting home from work – not always possible when kids are involved. The evening arsenic hours of 'bed, bath and beyond' exhaust most parents. These tasks are chores, to be sure, but keep participating in at least some of those activities or resentment will build and that's hard to come back from.

Tips for getting through the exam with a family:

- Take frequent short breaks during study to do a brief activity with your partner and kids. Physical activity is great, like kicking a football around or playing chase. This is great for your mental health and helps with study too.
- When you come back from work in the evening, the chores are done and the kids are in bed, just do MCQ-style study (see Chapter 6). The online MCQ-based resources are perfect for working parents.
- Study more intensively on days off and weekends. Set aside specific time to study that fits in with family activities. Use fun activities as a reward for a study session (e.g. 'I will study for an hour at 6.30, then take Lily to her soccer game' or 'I will study for two hours this afternoon while the kids watch the *Frozen* DVD for the millionth time then take them out for dinner while my partner goes for a bike ride').
- Listen to lectures (audio files or podcasts) on the way to and from work. I had all the audio files downloaded onto my iPhone and listened to them daily when I cycled to work.
- Watch lectures straight after work in the library before going home.
- Have frequent breaks from regular work by scheduling study days, and make the most of them.
- Ask for jobshare/part-time work prior to the exam. It works well for the Written because it gives you a lot of time to study at home when the kids are at school, but I would strongly recommend against doing it prior to Clinical exam! To prepare well for the Clinical, you have to be at the hospital as much as possible, as everything including acute admissions can be a perfect opportunity to practise examination skills, revise differentials and plan investigations and treatment.
- Routine family activities also help. I made sure that I watched kids' movies with them once a week and read them bedtime stories at least twice a week.

- Have proper, well-timed, relaxing holidays with the family. I went camping for five days with my family three weeks before the Written Exam and on a road trip for five days three weeks before the Clinical. I did not do any studying during that time which I think was beneficial as I managed to study very intensively for the two weeks immediately before the exams.
- Beware of really long holidays. I took six weeks off in August and went to the USA, Europe and Hong Kong with the whole family. Great trip, but my study group revved up, the hospital teaching was in full gear and I fell behind. I was rested and ready to study hard but I don't think that I ever caught up with my study group peers, which was especially noticeable during the two-week exam prep course. I would not recommend such long holidays in the middle of studying.
- I noticed that apart from brief but frequent quality breaks with my family, other non-study-related activities were relaxing and potentially beneficial for me. Our cleaner had to leave the country so we decided to do it ourselves and despite the initial dread, I actually found it relaxing. Similarly, the garden got to a point of severe neglect and I was forced to do some weeding, pruning and planting, which again proved to be a mindful and relaxing activity and seemed to increase my studying efficiency.
- Other people find a cleaner, online groceries and meal delivery to be a real time (and therefore study) saver. Try it out and see what works best for your family.
- Towards the end of my studying for the Written, I was eating more, sitting more and doing less physical activity. On went the kilos. My solution for that was that whenever I watched the online lectures, I would use wireless headphones and pace around the room, and do a few push-ups and sit-ups. I noticed that instead of it distracting me from the content of the lectures, it actually made me concentrate and absorb more. Some people are 'distractive learners' and this is how they learn – this definitely applies to me and might to you as well.
- For the Clinical Exam, the weekend Delta-Med course in Melbourne was inspiring, time efficient and changed my long case preparation for the better (see Chapter 13).
- The Clinical Exam was much harder on me and the family. I hardly spent any time at home for the last month and a half. I stayed until 6 or 7 pm every day after work. I was at the hospital at least one day of each weekend. I basically told my wife and kids that they would only see me for one hour a day and a few hours on the weekends.

The expectations were kept low and it went OK. The fact that we had holidays planned after the exam helped as we had something to look forward to as a family.

- I found it healthy and motivating to reward myself every now and then with a glass of wine or a movie in the evening once every couple of weeks. At times, cooking a meal for my family felt like a reward to me – like gardening, it felt like rest as it was mindful and relaxing.

On the whole, my family survived and so did I. The last six weeks before the Clinical were the hardest. I passed both the Written and Clinical Exams. I probably studied less than other people, but I think I studied more effectively and made the most of the time that I had.

33

Organising the Clinical Exam

You may wonder why on earth we thought a chapter on organising the FRACP Clinical Exam could be useful. Our reasons are twofold. First, inside knowledge of how the exam is organised helps candidates prepare, takes away some of the mystery and will calm your nerves on the day. Second, you may get roped into organising the Clinical Exam at your hospital at any stage in your career, a worthwhile and rewarding task that requires the patience of a saint and consumes a ridiculous amount of time, especially if you've never done it before and have to start from scratch.

First Principles

The FRACP Clinical Exam must be run with military precision. Precise time keeping is imperative to ensure the day runs smoothly. All participants (examiners, observers, patients and candidates) must be in the right place at the right time. This sounds easy, but remember that we are dealing with physicians and their registrars, known for rambling ward rounds, extended dithering and prolonged coffee breaks. Getting these folk to behave can be like herding cats, but must be done. Preparing to host the Clinical Exam begins before the Written Exam has taken place. Early organisation is crucial.

In New Zealand, the task of organising the exam is divided (like everything) into North and South, alternating each year. Auckland is so top-heavy population-wise that the dividing line is set at Palmerston North.

How to Pass the RACP Written and Clinical Exams: The Insider's Guide,
Second Edition. Zoë Raos and Cheryl Johnson.
© 2017 John Wiley & Sons Ltd. Published 2017 by John Wiley & Sons Ltd.

Organising the People and the Space

You need the right number of well-prepared staff leading up to the day and on Exam Day itself to help with myriad tasks that crop up. Start assembling your team of helpers in February. Nursing staff and administration staff are paid by the College for the time spent.

- **College staff members** – one or two staffies will be allocated to your centre. They are founts of knowledge and reassurance. At least one will have experience in running the exam and be full of institutional memory and on the day both will act as timekeepers and make sure the people-flow is on track. They will also help with catering so the examiners (who will eat loads of food), the candidates (who hardly eat anything) and everyone else is fed and watered.
- **Local registrar 'bulldogs'** – 'bulldogs' have been present in the Australian Clinical Exam. Pre-exam registrar helpers will become the norm in NZ soon. If you have the opportunity to be a 'bulldog', seize this fantastic chance to find out what this exam is all about before you are faced with doing it the next year. You may have wondered where the term 'bulldog' comes from … folklore suggests this term may have originated from the UK where the 'bulldog' was a member of the private police force at the University of Oxford.
- **Post-exam ATs** – choose two highly organised and efficient advanced trainees to help before and during the Clinical Exam. These registrars can find patients, help with all the phone calls and with traffic flow on the day. It is very useful for registrars to participate in exam organisation for all sorts of reasons.
- **Admin support whizz** – enlist a trusted departmental secretary or similar to keep track of all the paperwork before the exam and act as an extra pair of hands on the day. The paperwork is burdensome, and this particular support is invaluable.
- **Nursing staff/healthcare assistants** – depending on the number of candidates and cases, about three are required on the day to care for the patients, ensure they are appropriately prepared, are in the correct location and help them with toileting and other medical issues that invariably crop up.
- **Examiners** – these will be given to you by the College, and go through a rigorous process of calibration leading up to the day. You will almost certainly have some observers or 'provisional examiners'

who are working towards examiner status. The number of examiners will depend upon the number of candidates.

- **Candidates** – the number of candidates to be examined in your centre will be given to you by the College. This helps to work out how many cases you need to organise.
- **Clinic space** – get to know your clinic charge nurse, and advise them that a block of suitable rooms will need to be booked for Exam Day, and book them now. Generally, most centres will have been used in the past for the exam, but if not, contact your College staffies to advise how many clinic rooms will need to be booked, and also how many auxiliary rooms (separate holding areas for the examiners, candidates and patients). Most centres need at least three months' notice to ensure that clinics are not booked. Make sure there are plenty of available loos for nervous patients, candidates and examiners.

Case Selection Formula

The total number of cases needed = 2 × the number of candidates sitting at your centre. Using an imaginary Exam Day as an example, if you have 12 candidates, six short and long case patients are seen in the morning session (12 patients altogether), with the remaining six of each seen in the afternoon session (the last 12 patients). That means 24 patients in total – 12 × short cases and 12 × long cases. Each long case needs two rooms – one for the long case patient and one for discussion with the examiners. The table below illustrates the formula for other candidate numbers.

Candidates	Examiners	Long cases	Short cases	Exam rooms
8	8	8	8	12
12	12	12	12	18
16	16	16	16	24

Whilst many long case patients would be excellent short cases (and vice versa), this doesn't work on the day, so stick to the formula. The College will inform you of the number of candidates expected to be examined at your centre. At *least* two short and long case back-ups are needed for each session which is four back-ups in total (see more below on back-ups).

Types of Cases You Need to Find

Short Cases

Short cases are grouped to avoid confusion and to ensure that each candidate gets one each of the Big Three: a cardiology, a respiratory and a neurology. The fourth case can be anything – 'potluck'. Typically, cardiology and respiratory short cases are seen in the morning and neurology short cases are in the afternoon – the latter often have mobility issues, so an afternoon kick-off is easier logistically. The fourth 'potluck' cases will be a mixture of rheumatology, endocrine, gastroenterology or a repeat of the Big Three. When organising the actual sessions for the day, the candidates need a wide range of cases, *not* the examiners. If the examiners end up with a cardiology short case morning and afternoon that's not a problem … it is the candidates who need the variety for a fair exam.

Long Cases

Long cases are not grouped but a wide range of primary problems is advisable across the cases you choose. Some conditions may be similar between patients but candidates should not receive two 'diabetes-focused' or 'renal dialysis-focused' patients for fairness, so keep this in mind when organising the actual sessions on the day. The case-mix will depend a lot on what patients are seen in your hospital. It is a good idea to get one of each of the following for your cohort of patients (plus extras).

- Organ transplant (heart, liver, renal, lung, small bowel)
- End-stage renal failure on dialysis (CAPD, haemodialysis, waiting for transplant)
- Complicated diabetes
- HIV infection
- Rheumatoid arthritis or scleroderma
- Congestive heart failure or cardiomyopathy
- Complicated liver disease or inflammatory bowel disease
- Chronic neurological disease, e.g. CIDP or MND
- Long-term steroid use

> **Paeds Point**
>
> Organising the paediatric exam represents the next level of super-human skill. You will be organising children of all sizes, their parents and their families. Child patients travel great distances to get to clinic appointments and also to the exam. Parents may require childcare for remaining siblings at home. You will need to write notes excusing caregivers off work. All the things that can go wrong for the adult medicine exam can go even more pear-shaped for the paediatric exam. Thankfully, the actual number of candidates per exam centre is manageable, and there will be good institutional memory from past exam organisers to tap into.
>
> **Good long cases to find**
>
> - Transplant – liver, renal, cardiac, lung
> - Chronic kidney disease/dialysis/transplant
> - Epilepsy
> - Life-threatening asthma
> - ADHD
> - Autism spectrum disorder
>
> **Common short cases**
>
> - Congenital cardiac disease
> - Rheumatic heart disease
> - Cystic fibrosis
> - Neurodevelopmental

Where Are Cases Found?

You need to canvas/harass/hound all general and subspecialty physicians at your centre for exam patients starting in February, with ongoing reminders/arm twisting/endless group emails until you have *way more* than the required number of patients by March. As the emails come in, enter each patient in your (password protected to your institution's privacy requirements) Master Exam Excel Spreadsheet to keep track of which patients are confirmed. The College also gives you another spreadsheet which includes candidates, patients and examiners and is the 'mind-map' spreadsheet for where everyone should be on the day.

These are the suggested headings for that spreadsheet:

Name, NHI number	Contact details (mobile, home, email, address)	Short case or long case	System	Brief summary	AM or PM session	Letter sent	Taxi or travel by car	Confir-mation

Start contacting all patients in early April, and brace yourself for rejection. Weddings, funerals, bar mitzvahs, Pacific cruises, unwell spouses and pet vaccinations could stand in the way of a full cohort of patients on the day.

Confirm your Master Patient List in May, at least one month prior to the exams, by telephoning each patient. If possible, try to examine each patient yourself, for example during an inpatient stay or ask if you can pop into their next outpatient appointment to confirm physical signs and suitability. Each centre has a cohort of famous patients who are kind enough to be examined year after year, so have a look at your predecessor's Master Patient List for inspiration.

Each short case patient is seen four times during the session and each long case patient is seen twice. Patients need to be robust enough to cope with this.

Once patients have been contacted by phone and have agreed to participate, a letter is sent to them with the exam details. The College provides a template letter. Patients should be encouraged to arrive by taxi, which is arranged by the local organiser (you) with the help of your administrator. Patients can arrive by car and are provided with petrol vouchers and parking cards at the end of the exam. All patients must be contacted during the week of the exam to confirm attendance and travel arrangements. We advise that you adjust your clinical work by cancelling clinics, swapping out of call and getting special leave for all/part of the week before the exam as you will be busy. Most patients are complete professionals, know when to turn up despite incredible disability and disease, and need minimal assistance. Some will require daily reassuring phone calls and careful co-ordination with hairdresser appointments.

Short Case Patients

Short case patients need to have clinical signs although they may be static or burnt out. There are always 'urban legends' of candidates seeing normal patients with no clinical signs. It should never be the intention of the local organiser to have such patients but this can occur if a patient fails to arrive and there are inadequate back-ups. As above, it is the expectation from the College that each candidate gets a cardiology, a respiratory, a neurology and a 'potluck' case so depending on the numbers of candidates, use this formula when confirming your cases. Of course, this formula can be thrown out the window when your mitral regurgitant and aortic sclerotic pull out on the morning, and need to be replaced from the ranks, so the well-prepared candidate must anticipate any permutation of cases.

Long Case Patients

All long case patients need to be able to provide a history and have decent physical signs. It is not advisable in adult cases to have a patient who requires a support person to give a history due to cognitive issues. Again, examiners and candidates need to be prepared to wheel out some cognitive testing for a patient with possible dementia, but this is rare. There is such a range of suitable long case patients that it is difficult to summarise (please see Chapter 15) but a good guide is listed above. They key thing for the exam organiser is that the patient has a high likelihood of turning up on the day and has many interesting medical and social issues for the examiners and candidates to discuss.

Back-Up Patients

All long and short case patients are seen by the examiners before each morning/afternoon session begins, and cases will be (gently) rejected if they are not appropriate. They might be too unwell on the day, or the signs may have vanished, or they may withdraw consent. This is where your back-ups come in. Patients need to be brought in from your back-up list in the event that a patient is not appropriate.

The most ideal back-up patient is one who can 'swing both ways' and be both a short or a long case.

The other important task for the week prior to the exam is to bolster your back-up list with suitable inpatients. Ask local registrars and practice examiners for suitable short and long cases from inpatients, examine them quickly and ask their consent to be back-up cases on the day. Add them to your Master Excel Exam Spreadsheet. For example, there might be someone on the inpatient waiting list for an aortic valve replacement or a patient with Parkinson's awaiting rehabilitation so be nice to them and feed them lots of appropriate snacks while they wait. Your back-up and back-up back-up patients are gold, don't be offended if some of your preorganised cases pull out at the last possible moment or are rejected by the examiners.

The Envelopes

In the weeks leading up to the exam, prepare a clinical summary of each case for the examiners. Long cases need a brief problem list and an accurate medication list. Examiners review the patients blind – one takes a history and examines the patient while the other takes notes. After 40 minutes with the patient, the examiners review the envelope summaries and relevant investigations. All short cases need a brief summary of all clinical signs along with a suggested stem. Examiners review the patient first followed by the provided information before writing their own stem.

As well as the clinical summary, the envelopes should include printed copies of investigations. Investigations should include blood tests, ECGs, radiology reports, lung function tests and echocardiogram data if available. Radiology slides are an important part of short and long case discussions, and are best put onto a PowerPoint presentation to show candidates, as rifling through the hospital intranet site is frustrating for examiners and candidates alike. Radiology should be relatively easy to interpret and CT/MRI scans should be one slice and be the 'money shot'. If PowerPoint slides are not an option, then print out high-resolution large-sized individual 'money shot' pictures. If you are using PowerPoint to review radiology, talk to your friendly IT geek to get a generic log-in for the clinic computers that does not time out or require the examiners to put in a password. There is nothing more irritating and time wasting than having to find the password when the computer has gone to sleep.

'Mind-Map' and Other Spreadsheets

In addition to your Master Exam Excel Spreadsheet, you also need your 'mind-map' spreadsheet for lining up the correct number of patients and planning and keeping track of all patients, candidates, examiners and rooms. Who will be where, who will be examining whom, and so on. There will need to be signs on each door, with a route map of where each room is and what is going on.

Let us imagine you are in a small centre, with four candidates. The patients stay put. The examiners and the candidates move around with the help of you and your team. This might be a timetable for the day:

Morning session

Candidate A	Candidate B	Candidate C	Candidate D
Long case W Liver transplant	Short case 1 Cardio	Long case X Diabetes	Short case 2 Respiratory
Long case W Discussion	Short case 2 Respiratory	Long case X Discussion	Short case 1 Cardio
Short case 1 Cardio	Long case W Liver transplant	Short case 2 Respiratory	Long case X Diabetes
Short case 2 Respiratory	Long case W Discussion	Short case 1 Cardio	Long case X Discussion
Lunch	Lunch	Lunch	Lunch

Afternoon session

Candidate A	Candidate B	Candidate C	Candidate D
Long case Y Lymphoma	Short case 3 RA hands	Long case Z Crohn's disease	Short case 4 Spastic gait
Long case Y Discussion	Short case 4 Spastic gait	Long case Z Discussion	Short case 3 RA hands
Short case 3 RA hands	Long case W Lymphoma	Short case 4 Spastic gait	Long case Z Crohn's disease
Short case 4 Spastic gait	Long case W Discussion	Short case 3 RA hands	Long case Z Discussion
End	End	End	End

Just when you thought you had enough spreadsheets … you need one more! All patient travel needs to be recorded on a spreadsheet supplied by the College. The College reimburses the taxi company directly so there is no need to send taxi chits. All patients coming by car get their petrol vouchers and parking tickets when they leave the venue but the College needs to know how many vouchers to supply.

The Day Before

Check your back-up back-up inpatients are still in hospital and are OK to be brought to the exam centre in case of emergency. Your main job will be answering the phone as the outpatient cases call, ask if you can babysit the dog (no), check their appointments for the tenth time (be nice) and ask when their taxi is due to arrive (reassure). Double-check the catering and that all your helpers are lined up. If not, recruit helpers to cover. The College staffies are total professionals and will help you to ensure someone is nominated to keep time.

On the Day

Get a strong coffee. Have several copies of the Master Exam Excel Spreadsheet plus the mind-map spreadsheet printed out for the support team. If you can print in colour that makes the spreadsheet pretty but also helps to colour code the patients/candidates/examiners. Have your mobile phone on and charged in case a patient pulls out. Get there nice and early. Arrange to meet the College staffies, your admin support whiz and the registrar helpers to outline the plan for the day and make sure everyone knows their responsibilities (the College staffies are particularly good at this). Make sure the catering is delivered. Nominate a team member to meet and greet the patients, check them off against the Master Exam Excel Spreadsheet and get them all to the correct rooms with the right envelopes. The examiners will do the rest. After the session, ensure the patients are happy and thank them for their time.

What Examiners Tell the Patients

Before the candidates enter the room, the examiners counsel the patients regarding the information they should provide. Patients are told *not* to withhold information and to answer questions honestly.

If the question is too personal or the patient does not wish to answer the question, they can decline the examiners and the candidates. Whether the patient chooses to disclose information being asked is part of the joy and unpredictability of the exam, and tests the examiners' and candidate's interview skills and ability to establish rapport. Patients can be rejected if there is too much difficulty obtaining a history. If the examiners have problems getting information, this forms part of the long case discussion and will be taken into account when marking candidates.

Can you see how easily your lovely plans can be disturbed by recalcitrant historians, traffic snarl-ups and guide dogs with diarrhoea? Despite our paranoia, with good help and organisation, the Clinical Exam will go ahead and run on time. This is real life, and disasters can and will happen (cardiac arrests, unstable angina and haematemesis have all reportedly occurred). It is up to you, your team, the examiners and the candidates to manage the patients and each other just as you do every day at work. For those fortunate enough to organise the exam, early preparation is key. You've done the hard work. You will get as little sleep the night before the exam as the candidate but for different reasons!

Summary

- You will need to run this exam with military precision. Start getting ready well before the Written Exam starts.
- If someone in your centre has organised the exam before, get as much information from them as possible, including cases used in the past.
- Get your team of experts lined up early: College staff, admin whizz, nursing staff and registrar helpers.
- Book the physical space where the exam will be held.
- Use every contact you have to find patients. You will need to be persistent.
- Make a Master Exam Excel Spreadsheet of potential patients. As the exam draws ever closer, confirm patients and back-up patients, including travel.
- Aim for the correct proportion of cases, and organise them across the rooms so each candidate has a fair mix of cases.
- Prepare envelopes for each case the week before.
- Be prepared for all kinds of disasters as best you can, including back-up patients.

34

Preparing for Your Medical Interview

Introduction

In the recent past, house officers drifted into training in medicine by default while their surgically inclined colleagues sweated for weeks over interviews. Medical registrars were invited to basic training by shoulder tapping and a nod from the Director of Physician Education. Interviews, when they happened, had a preordained conclusion involving nudges, winks and in-house politics. Those days are behind us. Medical students are pouring out of universities, with demand for training posts outstripping supply at every career stage. The modern medical student and junior doctor must expect and prepare for interviews from the get-go, and build on these skills year by year for pre-exam medical registrar positions, advanced training posts, non-training rotations in sought-after specialties and SMO posts. The best thing you can do for any interview is to think about it well in advance, give it the preparation it deserves and put yourself across professionally.

Medical school and working life as a doctor do not prepare you for job interviews. Speaking from personal experience, the skills needed in a career interview are very different from those needed in everyday working life as a doctor. When I was on maternity leave from my fellowship in Oxford, an SMO post at my preferred hospital in New Zealand was advertised. This was the job I'd always wanted but my brain was maternal mush. I thought back on my mediocre performance in a range of interviews over the years and shuddered. I had always hated interviews, but guffed my way through them and managed to get the jobs I wanted by my reputation as a hard-working

How to Pass the RACP Written and Clinical Exams: The Insider's Guide,
Second Edition. Zoë Raos and Cheryl Johnson.
© 2017 John Wiley & Sons Ltd. Published 2017 by John Wiley & Sons Ltd.

and enthusiastic doctor. To perform well in this interview for a proper boss job, I needed help. England answered.

The Brits are great at interviews. They are interviewed at every stage of their careers. There is an entire private industry for medical interviews. I was about to sign up for an expensive course in London, when one of my colleagues (who had just nailed a sweet job in tight competition) suggested I save my money and recommended a simple and inexpensive online interview skills course: www.medicalinterview preparation.co.uk/. I did it over four weeks in small chunks. The course completely changed how I think about interviews. When *How to Pass* needed updating, I asked what 'the people' wanted, and 'the people' (registrars) all wanted to know how to do better in their interviews. I emailed the guy who wrote the online course to invite him to write a chapter, and he did. Thanks Nalin. Cheryl and I have added some local flavour.

Oh, and I got the job.

While the online course is Brit-centric, 90% of the material is directly applicable to the Antipodes. There is free material available on Nalin's website which is valuable and useful. If you choose to do it, the online course is inexpensive and covers everything from getting your application and covering letter right, through to the interview itself. To keep it snappy, this chapter focuses on specific skills you can work on right now to improve your medical interview performance.

Chapter Author: Dr Nalin Wickramasuriya, Consultant Paediatrician, Queen Alexandra Hospital, Portsmouth, UK

Congratulations, You've Got an Interview!

Mixed feelings are common when you're called for an interview. Part of you will feel excited that people have rated your CV and covering letter. Part of you will dread that you will be tested and compared against other people. You may think back on previous interviews, where you've left the room thinking 'I can't believe I forgot to talk about my audit or team skills' or 'Gee, if I'd opened my mouth a bit wider I could have fitted my other foot in. I'm going to the pub'.

There are some very specific traps that doctors tend to fall into when faced with an interview. Let's explore some of the common pitfalls, and provide practical steps to help avoid them and achieve success. We will refer to 'the employer' to cover the broad range of possible people who could interview you.

Trap Number 1 – Giving a Straight Answer to a Straight Question

Solution: Respond to the Question and Sell Your Skills

Throughout our training, we have been drilled to give straight answers to straight questions. This is useful for clear and accurate communication.

Q 'What is the haemoglobin?'
A '65'
Q 'What are the co-morbidities?'
A 'Severe COPD. Acute kidney injury. Critical AS. Dementia.'
Q 'Do you really think a colonoscopy is a good idea?'
A 'No.'

Straight answers to straight questions help us develop deductive thinking, which we use to formulate differential diagnoses and management plans every day. Straight answers to straight questions will destroy you in an interview setting should *never answer* interview questions. You must *respond* to the question in a way that allows you to pursue the three goals you must achieve in your covering letter, CV and (crucially) your interview.

The Three Goals of an Interview

Rapport

1) **Gain Rapport** Dress, speak and act in a way that encourages the interview panel to like you. They are more likely to rate you higher. It's human nature. If the panel have an impression that the candidate is good, they will judge the candidate in a relatively positive way. This judgement happens in singing competitions, the Clinical Exam and in your interview. Encourage the panel to accept you into their 'club'. Be professional and polite. Maintaining eye contact

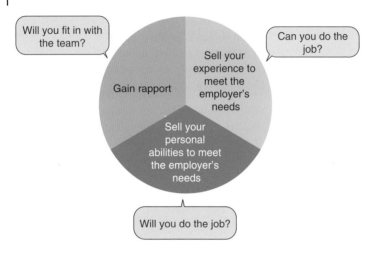

The Three Goals of an Interview

and a high smile rate are two body language traits that consistently correlate with a positive outcome at interviews. See Chapter 13 for what to wear to the Clinical Exam and make a sincere effort to look smart and conservative for any interview.

2 & 3) **Selling your Experience and Abilities** For these goals, know what skills you are selling and how to sell them. There are two sales strategies that are useful in interviews – the two Ss. The first is to **stress** the benefits of your skill, experience or knowledge. The second is to **show** your skills. As Katherine Mansfield said of short story writing, 'Always show, never tell'.

To stress the benefits of your skills, use language patterns to focus on how you can help the patients, the department and the hospital. Use sentences that start with:

- Having ...
- As a result of ...
- Because of ...

For example:

- Having worked for seven years in eight different general medicine departments, I feel confident looking after a wide range of patients at your hospital.

- As a result of completing my diploma in medical education, I think I can make a meaningful contribution to the training you offer here.
- Because of the research work I have done at the university, I feel that I can improve the ability of this unit to produce more translational research.

The next step is to add scenarios and real stories as evidence of your skills.

It is standard for medics to parrot statements in interviews:

- I am a team player
- I have excellent communication skills
- I am always patient focused.

These statements are repetitive and meaningless. Instead, use real stories to show how you are a team player with excellent communication skills and patient focus. Employ clever Jedi mind tricks to stand out from the crowd.

If you are going to tell a story, consider using the STAR structure for your response.

- **Situation** – Last year I was called in to see an acutely unwell decompensated alcoholic patient with haematemesis.
- **Task** – I needed to assess if the patient was a transplant candidate, resuscitate, arrange an urgent scope and find the next of kin.
- **Action** – I called the gastroenterology consultant. We established the patient was not a transplant candidate. When the patient went to theatre for the scope, I called in the family for an urgent meeting. It was difficult, as the patient had a young family with complex dynamics and they were angry and divided.
- **Result** – Over the next two days, I maintained close communication with the family. Through regular meetings and careful listening, I conveyed complex information in a way they were all able to understand. I worked closely with the gastroenterologist and the ward nurses to deliver the most appropriate care possible in a dynamic team setting. Unfortunately, the patient died of overwhelming sepsis and encephalopathy, peacefully, with his family around him. It was a tragic case, nonetheless I learnt a great deal about the local protocols for cirrhotic patients as well as the importance of meticulous communication across the board. I believe I can bring such skills to Christchurch Hospital as a gastroenterology advanced trainee.

What does the interview panel think? Wow, this person will fit in with us. This person can definitely do the job of a gastroenterology registrar. This person is passionate, and wants to do the job. Boom!

Trap Number 2 – The Short Case/Viva Complex

Solution: Manage Yourself and You Will Manage the Interview

Most of us have been tested in a short case, OSCE or viva setting during our medical training. That process has set up some deep-seated, heart-palpitating, hand-sweating psychological conditioning that can trigger inappropriate responses in an interview setting.

In an average short case or viva, the examiner is trying to work out what we don't know. The candidate senses danger and answers the question defensively. The aim is to get out alive, avoid digging holes, not look stupid and avoid failure. When we are faced with a 'grilling' from a consultant on a ward round, we often adopt the same mindset, which can often lead to dull and defensive answers.

Defensiveness and dullness are the enemies of a good interview. You must develop the confidence to control, manage and own the interview – your interview! Those excellent skills from managing your high-maintenance boss and wheedling a scan out of a radiology registrar are what to employ. You need to be able to move the topic of conversation to areas where you are strong – an interview is more of a two-way process than a viva. The interviewers aren't looking to find out what you don't know; they are looking to see what you can do, what you do know and if you could be a good fit for their department. They are approaching this differently and so should you. Be confident to manoeuvre discussion to areas of strength and experience. By preparing ahead, you will be able to plug your skills and experience into a response for any question.

Trap Number 3 – Preparing for the Interview Like an Exam

Solution: Think Ahead and Sell Your Skills and Experience

Some candidates can wing an interview without preparation and nail it – some are naturally gifted, some don't have strong competition. If you aren't naturally gifted at talking or if the post you are applying for is in demand, then you should prepare. But don't prepare for it like an exam.

As doctors, when we are stressed, we go looking for facts, it's just in our DNA. We did well at exams, this made us keener to study and qualify as doctors – a career-perpetuating self-fulfilling cycle of learning facts. When we get stressed, we go back to what we're good at – learning facts and regurgitating them. In interviews, we might talk about a review article, or p-values, or big trials that have come out of the specialty. An interview is not an exam and the interview panel have all the facts. The panel want to know… Can you do the job? Will you do the job? Will you fit in?

The key to doing well at an interview is to think ahead. You must out-think the interview panel and out-think your competition. Remember your goal of selling your skills to meet their needs? It's important that you understand what the patients, the department and the hospital that you are applying for need and want. Read the job description carefully. Do research about the department and the hospital. Read between the lines. If there is no detailed job description, then talk to a current registrar in that post and find out about the average working week and on-call responsibilities. Find out about training in the area, and what it involves.

By listening, reading and thinking about what the patients, department and hospital want and need, you can establish their 'buying' buttons. Once you know the real judgement criteria, then you will be better positioned to push those buttons through your answers. If you know that the hospital needs to provide a more streamlined service, talk about how you can help them to become more efficient. If you know the hospital is not up to scratch in a particular area, mention how you can assist them to improve their service.

It's important that you spend time thinking about your skills and experiences, and specifically how these relate to the job you are applying for. Think back to your training, and come up with specific examples that showcase your abilities. Google commonly asked interview questions, then write down responses and stories that sell the skills you have.

It is also important to come up with your own 12-month, five-year and 10-year career plans. This seems corporate and unphysicianly, but do it anyway. You will be answering many questions about your future on the day, know what you want your life to be like and be genuine and forthright in your responses.

Trap Number 4 – Talking Posh on the Day of the Interview

Solution: Be Personal, Specific and Honest

A common temptation is to use complicated sentences with big words in your interview to make you sound clever or more important. Resist at all costs!

The best answers have three features – they are personal, specific and honest.

Your default grammatical person should be the first person singular. Keep the topic of conversation about you and not doctors in general. Be specific in the content of your answers. By providing specific information or views, you will add credibility to your answers. By being vague and general, your answers will be perceived as dull and naive.

Be honest in your language. Say your stuff your way. Talk like you would normally talk – without the slang and swear words. At its core, an interview is a business meeting. So conduct yourself as you would at a formal handover or multidisciplinary meeting. Be honest in your content. Any fibs or fudging can be found out with reference checks – it just isn't worth it.

Your answers need to be about 2–3 minutes long. Any shorter and you risk missing chances to sell more skills. Any longer and you might put the panel to sleep!

You should look to structure your answers with an introduction, the 'guts' bit and conclusion. In the beginning, briefly answer the question and then introduce the structure of the body of your answer. In the body, focus on 2–4 themes. Be personal and specific and try to spend time explaining how you can help the patients, the department and the hospital. Conclude your answers by handing over speaking responsibility to the interviewer. Add value to your responses by showing – not telling.

Q   Why is clinical audit important?

A   Audit improves quality. For example, last year at St Elsewhere Hospital the bacteraemia rates from peripheral IV lines increased, which generated negative publicity. I worked with the infectious diseases team to audit aseptic non-touch technique for IV line insertion. We established the current rates of IV line-associated bacteraemia, then I developed an intervention plan including training sessions for doctors and nurses. There was resistance at first so I brought lollies along to the teaching sessions and made completion certificates for the participants. I re-audited IV line bacteraemia rates six months later, and they had dropped by 45%. I received consistent feedback that the educational sessions were practical and helpful. The nurses really liked the certificates for their portfolios. I presented this work in poster form at the national meeting, and got a prize for best clinical poster. Over 40 cases of IV line bacteraemia were prevented in a 12-month period, which is great news for these patients as far less morbidity, and positive for the hospital in reduced inpatient days. So, in summary, my project demonstrates the importance and usefulness of audit in a clinical setting and how it is important to get the whole team on board to make a positive change. I believe I can bring these skills and experience as an advanced infectious diseases trainee.

Trap Number 5 – Not Planning Your Response When the Interviewer Asks You a Question

Solution: Listen. Engage Brain. Structure Your Response

It's important to plan your responses. You always start a medical procedure with plan A or plan B, so in an interview don't start talking until a plan is hatched in your mind. Listen to the question, close your mouth, engage your brain and then answer.

To plan your answer, spend a few seconds thinking through the answers to three planning questions.

- What's this question really about?
- What skills and experience will I sell in response to this question?
- Which structure will I choose?

So make sure you listen carefully to the question, as it's really easy to answer the question you thought you heard or wanted to hear. Try to work out what's really being questioned – hint: it's likely to be about you. Figure out if the question is future based or past based. If the question is future based, then spend 80% of your time responding about what you would do in the future, which is where your career plan preparation comes in really handy. If the question is past based, then spend 80% of your time explaining what you have done and learnt in the past.

Then think about all the things that you could talk about in this question. You need to cast your net of ideas as wide as you can, so that you don't miss the chance to mention something that makes you look good, including being a team leader, fitting in well with others, showing initiative or some research you've done.

Next, figure out how you want to structure the answer. If it's a story, then use the STAR structure. Otherwise, consider using a nominative structure, where you will just name three things or themes. If you listen carefully to the root question word, then the structure will become apparent.

- If the question is Why, then talk about three reasons.
- If the question is How, talk about three ways.
- If the question is Who, talk about three groups of people.
- If the question is What, talk about three things.

There is even more to learn about interviews. We hope that awareness of the Five Traps will at least get you on the right track. If you are interested, have a look at Nalin's online course.

Summary

- Face your fear of medical interviews. Through preparation, you can be confident, sell yourself (without selling your soul) and stand out from the crowd.
- Beware of the five pitfalls that many doctors fall into. Know the solutions.
- Instead of answering a question, you must respond to it with specific examples that demonstrate your skills and experience.
- Can you do the job? Will you do the job? Will you fit in? These are the questions you must constantly ask and answer in your preparation, and on the day.
- Be prepared.

35

Career Planning

I Passed. What Advanced Training Programme Should I Apply For?

There are some registrars with a laser-like career focus. Those who knew that they wanted to be a neurologist from birth, who carried a natty green doctor's bag to the sandpit and could augment ankle jerks by the age of four. If this is you, your future is already mapped out.

Then, there's a moderately sure group of registrars, with a pretty good idea about what career path to take or who have narrowed it down to a couple of options. They ask around amongst like-minded advanced trainees and consultants well before the exam and have an idea when the interviews are.

Then, there's everyone else. Most Australian trainees are organised and well differentiated by the time the Written Exam comes along, whereas many Kiwis feel like an embryonic stem cell. We admire those who have a clear career path. But can we also say that there is nothing wrong with being pluripotent. It is OK to know you want to be a paediatrician or physician, and to not be sure about a specialty. Even at the post-exam stage. It is also very OK (more than OK, in fact) to aspire to be a general physician or paediatrician. We salute the generalists, the hardest job of all. If you do want to specialise, you need to be smart about it. And quick smart in New Zealand as, before you have even had time to breathe after the Clinical Exam, advanced training interviews will be upon you.

There is not room in this small tome to list every possible subspecialty, its advantages and disadvantages, the truth about advanced

How to Pass the RACP Written and Clinical Exams: The Insider's Guide, Second Edition. Zoë Raos and Cheryl Johnson.
© 2017 John Wiley & Sons Ltd. Published 2017 by John Wiley & Sons Ltd.

training, which hospitals have the best training and how likely a specialist trainee is to get a consultant job at the end of it. Some specialties, especially in larger centres, demand postgraduate degrees, PhDs and overseas fellowships of their advanced trainees before a consultant post can be offered so you'll need to do your homework. Advanced training will be over before you know it. Decisions you make now will have a big impact not only on the next few years of advanced training, but on your whole working life as a consultant.

Pearls of Wisdom

You will be a consultant much longer than you were a registrar. Depending on your age, you could be a rhubarbologist for 30 years. Choose a specialty that piques your interest academically, that has the type of patients that you like, that you can handle the dross of (and every specialty has its dross, just different types of subspecialised dross!) and has colleagues that you get on with and fit in with. This is not a popularity contest, but it sure helps being in a specialty of like-minded people when you're on a conference in Vancouver and need dinner company, or when you are really stuck with an incredibly complicated patient and need to ask your colleagues for help.

Choose a specialty where the work-life balance of the consultant you aspire to be fits in with the way you want to live your life. This is really important for everyone, not just for those with a family (or who one day might want to have a family). Be honest about your career aspirations, and balance these carefully against all the other aspects of your life. Work isn't always everything.

Advanced training in some specialties is notoriously awful. Extremely long hours, demanding patients and prima donna bosses make the Clinical Exam look like a walk in the park. Other training schemes are (in comparison) a doddle with very little on-call. Make sure that if you are going to endure hardship in training, the consultant job at the end of it is really what you want to do.

Think about the type of work-week you want when you are a consultant. Do you like ward rounds, relatively well patients, procedures, outpatient clinics or a bit of everything? Think about your current job and what you really love (and detest) about it. Do you like multidisciplinary meetings, end-of-life care, complex challenging patients/families, dealing with ICU? Do you want to have a private practice or remain within the confines of the hospital? Life as a consultant is quite different from that of a training registrar. Some specialties are heavy on outpatient clinics, others have a higher inpatient burden, some have chronic patients you get to know well. Some specialties rely on a functional multidisciplinary team of which the specialist consultant is the leader, other specialists are lone wolves by comparison.

May we suggest to the **undecided trainee**: sign up for advanced training in general and acute care medicine or general paediatrics. Then, any time you spend post exam will count towards something highly worthwhile.

If you are interested but undecided on a specialty, send in your application, turn up for the interview (see Chapter 35), prepare for it and be honest. Say that you want a job to see if the specialty is a mutual fit. Most decent specialty interview panels are understanding of advanced trainees who are making career decisions and may even have non-training posts for such registrars. An undecided advanced trainee is still a great asset to have on the team. Your job in the interview is to convince them of this.

Career Path Planning

Once you know what you want to do, and get accepted, getting your career path sorted out is tricky, nebulous and complicated compared to the prescribed path of plodding through basic training and the exams. Some specialties have well-trodden advanced training programmes. Others you organise yourself, with little guidance. There are many different ways to dual train, to train across different centres, to change specialties and to train with another colleges for more exam fun. Seek advice from mentors, senior registrars and consultants. Go through the College training requirements and do as much planning as you can right from the start and work out the runs you want to complete. Make sure you're up to date with all your paperwork requirements and consider all your options for training.

Once you complete advanced training, the fun is not over. Organising fellowships, higher degrees and finding a consultant job can be even more heart-wrenching and nightmarish. Someone should write a book about it!

Get a Mentor

A final and important note ... get a mentor. Consider getting more than one. Different mentors are useful for different things. An exam mentor might be a registrar from the next year up who passes on notes and keeps your spirits up. A career mentor might be a consultant you've always got on with in the specialty you are interested in, who can arrange formal and informal meetings for career progress. Some career mentors are those you see at morning tea, not always in the specialty you want to join, who offer unbiased advice and are well connected. It can be useful to have a mentor for balancing life outside medicine who understands the particular situation you face every day, such being a parent, being an athlete, being gay, being from a particular ethnic group, being a musician, being in recovery from addiction ... someone who can understand and give support throughout your career. Hopefully, you too will become a mentor to others – it takes up little time but is an immensely rewarding exercise.

Summary

- It is big career decision time. It is OK to know exactly what you want to do and it is OK to have a rough idea. It is OK to have no idea. You will need a clear strategy for the next 12–24 months irrespective of your decision.
- When deciding on a specialty, think carefully about life and work as a consultant in that specialty.
- Do reconnaissance on the perils of an advanced training pro-gramme – are you up for it? Is it worth it?
- If you're not sure of your exact career trajectory, it really is OK. Enrol in general paediatrics or general medicine so your time will count while you decide.
- Prepare for interviews.
- During and after advanced training, plan your career path using careful thinking and advice.
- Get a mentor or two. They are highly useful people to have in your life. Be a mentor to others. It's a great system.

36

OK, We'll Stop Talking Now!

Both the Written and Clinical Exams will stand out as suitably traumatic events in our lives. The hours of study and angst that we suffered were legion, and much support was gleaned from those who waded through the pain with us. The writing of the first edition of this book was cathartic and healing (feel free to write your own book if you want to treat your own post-traumatic stress disorder) and updating the second edition took us back to the pain. We hope this new edition will help the next generation of FRACP candidates, just as the first edition helped many who are now consultants.

In the course of writing this book and updating it, we cornered lots of registrars and consultants over morning tea and nagged them for their input. Most people said roughly the same thing.

- The examiners have to pass someone. With hard work and the right approach, that someone could be you.
- The exams are horrible but you can survive them. One way or another, the exams will come and go, and you will get your life back.
- If you fail, you most certainly are not the first good doctor to do so. Take heart and believe in yourself. There is always next year.
- If you pass, fantastic! You can move on to the challenges of advanced training and show others (drum roll ...) how to pass.

We hope this book will make this rite of passage bit easier for you than it was for us. We wish you all the very best of luck.

How to Pass the RACP Written and Clinical Exams: The Insider's Guide, Second Edition. Zoë Raos and Cheryl Johnson.
© 2017 John Wiley & Sons Ltd. Published 2017 by John Wiley & Sons Ltd.

Helping the Next Lot

If you want to help the next lot of registrars, please email us any pearls of wisdom you acquired on your journey. We would also appreciate your opinion on glaring errors or omissions. Let us know what you think and we'll try and put it all in the next edition of *How to Pass*! zoe_raos@yahoo.co.nz

Index